HEALTH PROBLEMS IN DOWN SYNDROME

Edited by **Subrata Dey**

Health Problems in Down Syndrome
http://dx.doi.org/10.5772/59349
Edited by Subrata Dey

Contributors

Shannon Ringenbach, Subrata Kumar Dey, Cristina Areias, Benedita Sampaio-Maia, Viviana Macho, Ana Norton, Paula Macedo, Casimiro Andrade, Fatma Soylemez, Masayuki Yamamoto, Jumana Al-Aama

Published by InTech

Janeza Trdine 9, 51000 Rijeka, Croatia

Publishing Process Manager Iva Simcic

Technical Editor InTech DTP team

Cover InTech Design team

First published September, 2015

Printed in Croatia

Additional hard copies can be obtained from orders@intechopen.com

Health Problems in Down Syndrome, Edited by Subrata Dey

p. cm.

ISBN 978-953-51-2154-1

For EU product safety concerns:
IN TECH d.o.o., Prolaz Marije Krucifikse Kozulić 3, 51000 Rijeka, Croatia,
info@intechopen.com or visit our website at intechopen.com.

Meet the editor

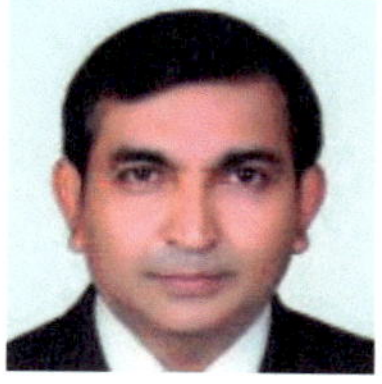

Dr. Subrata Dey is the Professor of Biotechnology and Pro-Vice Chancellor at Maulana Abul Kalam Azad University of Technology (formerly West Bengal University of Technology). His laboratory has long been involved in research on the molecular genetics of Down syndrome. His current research interests include the identification of genes involved in the development of congenital heart disease and Alzheimer's disease in both Down syndrome and healthy individuals. His group also studies the mechanism of radiation induced genomic instability and radioprotection. Prof. Dey has been teaching courses in genetics, molecular biology, and developmental biology for more than thirty years. Dr. Dey is the author of many research papers and has supervised research works of many students. He has also edited three books on Down syndrome. Prof. Dey is the founding director of the Centre for Genetic Studies and has developed a free online learning portal on genetics and genetic disorders (www.genomegyan.com).

Contents

Preface

This book focuses on research and review articles on common health problems associated with Down syndrome. Trisomy 21, commonly referred to as Down syndrome, is the most frequent live born aneuploidy in humans. Although several hypotheses have been suggested regarding the origin of trisomy 21 Down syndrome, the etiological factors are under continuous scrutiny since its discovery. Meiotic nondisjunction of chromosome 21 due to advanced maternal age and reduced recombination are identified as two strong correlates that affect proper segregation of chromosomes at oogenesis, particularly at first meiotic division. Moreover, the process of oogenesis is lengthy and involves meiotic arrests which makes it more vulnerable to malsegregation of chromosomes than spermatogenesis. It has been suggested that with increasing maternal age, there is a rapid degradation of cellular proteins involved in spindle formation and anaphase separation in oocytes, which imposes the risk of nondisjunction or nonseparation of chromosome both at first and second meiotic divisions. Down syndrome birth is also attributable to multiple maternal risk factors that include both genetic and environmental challenges. However, there is limited understanding of the complicated interaction among these factors. Periconceptional smoking, use of oral contraceptives, and chewing tobacco are some of the environmental risk factors identified in several epidemiologic studies on Down syndrome. Moreover, it has been suggested that the genetics that underlies nondisjunction of chromosome 21 is probably universal irrespective of racial differences across human population.

In addition to the intellectual and developmental disabilities, children with Down syndrome are at an increased risk for certain health problems. However, each individual with Down syndrome is different, and not every individual will have serious health problems. Many of these associated conditions can be treated with medication, surgical intervention, and regular exercise.

This book is organized into three sections. These sections include chapters on recent advances in research on health problems in Down syndrome.

Section I describes our present knowledge on different diseases associated with Down syndrome. Individuals with Down syndrome suffer from different types of diseases of which altered metabolism is attributable to the overexpression of some chromosome 21 genes. Risk for solid tumor is significantly reduced in Down syndrome. In contrast, Down syndrome children have increased risk of developing leukemia. Moreover, Down syndrome individuals have higher prevalence of periodontal diseases, which develop at early age. They can live full, productive, and quality lives with help from modern medicine, surgical intervention, and lifetime support program.

Section II deals with improvement of cognitive skills in Down syndrome. Exercise is a logical intervention for effective treatment for cognitive impairments in individuals with Down syndrome.

Section III presents articles on recent research approaches on Down syndrome. Down syndrome or trisomy 21 is one of the most important genetic causes of mental retardation. Sincere and significant attempts have been made towards understanding the congenital diseases that affect Down syndrome patients. Better understanding of gene networks associated with such malformations will help to predict the complex genetic trait behind congenital diseases in Down syndrome. It will also provide the basis for tailored gene therapies that could begin to heal or prevent such malformation without the need to resort to invasive surgery. Aneuploidy is the second most important category of chromosome mutation. It arises by nondisjunction of chromosome during meiosis. Characteristics of double aneuploidies in Down syndrome have also been reviewed.

This book provides a concise yet comprehensive source of current information on Down syndrome. All the articles are very interesting and provide up-to-date knowledge on recent progress in the area of common health problems in Down syndrome. This book is expected to serve as a reference work for research workers, scientists, medical practitioners, and health care providers.

The editor wants to acknowledge the superb assistance and support of the staff members and management of Intech Publishers, in particular, Ms. Iva Simcic for her coordination and editorial assistance. We gratefully acknowledge all contributing authors and scientists who made this book possible by providing valuable research and review articles.

Prof. Subrata Dey
Department of Biotechnology,
West Bengal University of Technology,
Kolkata, West Bengal, India

Section 1

Diseases Associated with Down Syndrome Indivuduals

Chapter 1

Altered Metabolism in Down Syndrome

Jumana Y. Alaama, Muhammad S. Ahmad,
Sultan Ahmad and Zoheir A. Damanhouri

Additional information is available at the end of the chapter

http://dx.doi.org/10.5772/60638

Abstract

Down syndrome (DS) is associated with aberrations in genetic, morphological, biochemical and physiological characteristics. A number of genes located on human chromosome 21 (HSA21) encode proteins which are thought to be involved in numerous metabolic pathways, e.g., phosphofructokinase, cystathionine β-synthase etc. Perturbations of the metabolic pathways may lead to altered drug metabolism in DS individuals. We present a review of metabolic aberrations linked to HSA21 genes in DS. We particularly focus on drug disposition, efficacy, sensitivity and toxicity of anti-leukaemic agents including methotrexate, glucocorticoids, anthracyclines and cytarabine in DS leukaemia. The different outcomes of therapy due to differential drug response, varied drug toxicity and treatment related mortality in DS leukaemia is a subject of much research and speculation. Altered drug response in DS individuals may stem from differences in pharmacokinetics, pharmacodynamics and pharmacogenetics. Further large-cohort studies in different age groups dissecting metabolic and molecular pathways involved in drug response may increase our understanding in this regard and stipulate pharmacotherapies in DS.

Keywords: Down Syndrome, Drug Metabolism, Pharmacokinetics, Pharmacodynamics, Methotrexate, Leukaemia, Glucocorticoids, Anthracyclines, Cytarabine

1. Introduction

Down syndrome (DS) is the most commonly reported genetic disorder characterized by intellectual disability which occurs in approximately 1/700 live births [1]. Despite advances in antenatal screening and pregnancy termination, the prevalence of DS is increasing due to advanced maternal age and increased longevity of DS individuals [2-4]. Trisomy of all or part of human chromosome 21 (HSA21) is the underlying genetic abnormality that causes DS. Some 200-300 genes have been identified to be located on the long arm as well as on a portion of the short arm of chromosome 21 in DNA sequencing studies [5]. The overexpression of such genes likely results in cascading effects, eliciting interactions among gene products and between genes and environmental factors. These cause aberrations in the morphological, biochemical and physiological milieu of DS individuals resulting in the characteristic manifestations of DS.

Down syndrome Individuals exhibit altered metabolism which is attributed to the overexpression of some HSA21 localized genes or due to the presence of extra genetic information. A number of genes located on HSA21 encode enzymes those are thought to be involved in numerous metabolic pathways such as inositol, energy, cholesterol, choline, purine and reactive oxygen species pathways [6]. In this chapter, we review the literature for characteristic metabolic aberrations linked to HSA21 genes in DS. We particularly focus on the efficacy of chemotherapeutic agents such as methotrexate, glucocorticoids, anthracyclines and cytarabine in the context of drug disposition, sensitivity and toxicity in DS individuals since these agents form the backbone of current anti-leukaemic therapies.

2. Gene-dosage effects

Several genes involved in metabolism are located on chromosome 21 such as cystathionine β-synthase (CBS) gene encoding the CBS enzyme that catalyses homocysteine into cystathionine. Due to the presence of an extra copy of CBS gene in DS individual, lower levels of homocysteine and methionine are found in DS individuals compared to normal people which in turn leads to folate shortage and an altered metabolic state. Formimidoyltransferase cyclodeaminase (FTCD) is another gene located on the long arm of chromosome 21 which provides instruction to produce formimimotransferase cyclodeaminase enzyme involved in the metabolism of histidine and the production of folate required for synthesis of purine, pyrimidines and amino acids. Variations in the activities of various enzymes and plasma electrolyte concentrations to differ from normal parameters in DS have previously been reported especially in HSA 21 associated proteins such as S100B [7]. The levels of S100B protein were 4-8 times higher in DS individuals compared to the reference values. In addition, changes in metabolism of adenosine, homocysteine, purine and folate have also been reported [6].

Phosphofructokinase (PFK) is a key regulatory enzyme in glycolytic pathway as it catalyses the phosphorylation of fructose-6-phospate to fructose-1, 6-bisphosphate [8]. Liver-type subunit of PFK (PFKL) is overexpressed in DS patients because its gene is located on chromosome 21 [9, 10]. Peled-Kamar *et al.* showed that transgenic mice overexpressing PFKL (Tg-PFKL) had aberrated glucose metabolism characterized by increases metabolic rate in brain and reduced clearance rate from the blood [11]. The enhanced glucose utilization observed in brain of Tg-PFKL mice is similar to faster cerebral glucose metabolism exhibited by young DS adults and may be linked to their cognitive disabilities. A previous study reported that PFK specific activity is increased two-fold in the brains of embryonic Tg-PFKL mice [12] highlighting the fact that aberration in glucose metabolism are more pronounced in developmental period and may lead to DS associated learning disabilities. This observation of differential gene expression at different developmental stages further complicates the hypothesis of 'gene-dosage effects' in trisomy 21 consequently leading to varied metabolism aberration among different age groups. Further studies to determine metabolic variations in different age groups will not only increase our understanding in this regard but will also stipulate pharmacotherapies in DS.

3. Drug metabolism in Down syndrome

The effect of perturbations in metabolic pathways in DS is also reflected in the area of drug metabolism. Altered drug response has been reported in DS individuals compared to normal people, which may stem from differences in pharmacokinetics (PK) and pharmacodynamics (PD) in DS. Drug metabolizing enzymes, especially cytochrome P450, are a major source of variability in the PK of drugs. The CYP3A subfamily is believed to metabolize half of all prescribed drugs. Differences in the activity of cytochrome P450 may explain the altered drug response in DS individuals. We studied the CYP3A4/5 activity and found that children with DS had a 2.4 fold lower CYP3A4/5 activity compared to the children without DS (unpublished data). Alterations in PD have been reported for opioids, midazolam, acetylsalicylic acid and atropine [6, 13]. The metabolism of drugs is known to influence the active drug concentration of a drug, which either boosts or causes a reduced action of that drug. A drug which is subjected to increased metabolism will have a diminished intensity of drug action, as an increased metabolism will limit its duration of activity. On the contrary, a decline in the metabolism of the drug will intensify drug activity. Down syndrome individuals have a lower resting metabolic rate compared to normal people, which may contribute to altered drug metabolism and drug toxicity. Gut microbial chemical messengers regulate and influence host metabolism. Differences in gut microbiome may also be a relevant factor in altered drug metabolism in DS individuals and a review of literature is needed in this regard.

Down syndrome children are known to have an approximately 10- 20 times higher risk of developing some blood cancers such as acute lymphoblastic leukaemia (ALL) and acute myeloid leukaemia (AML) compared to non-DS children [14, 15]. In the last two decades, numerous studies have identified various drugs showing altered metabolism in DS patients in the context of childhood leukaemias. For instance, DS children suffering from AML have a better prognosis over non-DS children with AML. An *in vitro* study showed that DS-AML myeloblasts exhibited ten times higher sensitivity towards 1-beta-D-arabinofuranosylcytosine (ara-C), compared to myeloblasts from non-DS AML children [16]. On the other hand DS children with ALL show a pronounced intolerance for methotrexate which necessitates dose reductions and further adjustments in treatment protocols.

As described above, DS individuals have a high risk of developing haematological conditions, of which the most prominent is the development of acute leukaemias [17]. Acute lymphoid leukaemia (ALL), acute myeloid leukaemia (AML) and a unique type of leukaemia exclusively associated with trisomy 21 called transient myeloproliferative disorder (TMD), commonly arise in DS individuals [18]. It has been recognized that while the presence of chromosome 21 trisomy on the one hand might be a deterrent against development of certain solid tumours in DS individuals, on the other hand it compounds the risk of development of haematological tumours [17]. Of note, is the fact that the acute leukaemias in DS shows marked differences from acute leukaemias in non-DS individuals. This varied picture reflects the underlying change, which ranges from molecular to systems level in DS individuals and confers unique characteristics to host and disease biology including marked differences in disease outcomes as compared to non-DS leukaemia patients. The different outcomes of therapy due to differential drug response, varied drug toxicity and treatment related mortality (TRM) remains in DS leukaemia a subject of much research and speculation. In this connection, various studies in the last two decades have highlighted the direct or indirect involvement of the extra copy of chromosome 21 with its gene dosage imbalances as a basic factor [19]. Additionally, acute leukaemia is known to be a highly heterogeneous disease [20, 21]. In DS patients with their characteristic biochemical and pathophysiological state it most likely contributes to the distinctive malignancy pattern observed in them.

Recent studies have identified new subtypes of DS leukaemia patients [22, 23]. The subtypes show distinctive prognostic features which also have a bearing on event free survival (EFS) rates. This brings into perspective the issue of present drugs commonly used for the treatment of leukaemia in DS, their metabolism and treatment outcomes. In this respect, studies linking the genes or possible candidate genes involved, the molecular pathways influenced by these genes, the gene products, the pathophysiologic milieu of DS leukaemia and the pharmacological differences emerging thereof have begun to clarify the drug sensitivity, drug responsiveness and drug toxicity profiles in the setting of DS leukaemia. This has resulted in protocol modifications in certain cases of DS leukaemia and improved treatment outcomes [24, 25]. Patients' response to a particular therapeutic regimen and the drugs concerned happens to be the most crucial prognostic predictor of treatment outcomes. In this context both malignant cell genetics and patients' pharmacodynamics and pharmacogenetics are intimately involved [26].

Studies in drug pharmacodynamics and pharmacokinetics have been helpful in informing and formulating treatment regimens in DS and NDS leukaemia patients. Pharmacogenetics and pharmacogenomics deals with the effect of a particular gene or genome wide associations respectively on drug response of an individual [27]. Pharmacogenomics is a relatively new and promising area which has the potential to unravel the enigmatic issues associated with DS leukaemia. Altered metabolism of drugs is well recognized in cancers including leukaemia and DS leukaemia [28-30]. High to severe drug related toxicity in ALLDS patients is a known phenomenon. The toxicities may be related to the gastrointestinal mucosa, infectious toxicity secondary to MTX use, haematological toxicity and hepatic toxicity, which under severe circumstances may lead to liver fibrosis and neurological toxicity [31]. Besides, ALLDS patients exhibit a higher level of resistance to certain drugs used in various chemotherapeutic regimens than ALLNDS individuals.

In DS individuals, more data are present for anti-leukaemic agents than any other drug. Therefore, we present a detailed review of methotrexate, glucocorticoids, anthracyclines and cytarabine in the next section.

4. Methotrexate

Methotrexate (MTX), an anti-folate agent [19] is one of the most widely used and frequently studied drugs in various malignancies including leukaemia [22]. In ALL, the drug is usually administered as high dose MTX (HDMTX) which constitutes 500mg/m^2 and above. It is an anti-metabolite that inhibits cellular growth by obstructing the formation of purines and thymidine phosphate. MTX is known as a competitive inhibitor of dihydrofolate reductase, (DHFR), an enzyme required for the conversion of terahydrofolate from dihydrofolate in dividing cells. MTX competitively binds to DHFR, replacing dihydrofolate. This results in the lack of regeneration of tetrahydrofolate, a reduced folate that is essential for de novo purine and thymidine phosphate synthesis. This eventually blocks DNA synthesis [32-34].

MTX entry into the cell is facilitated by the reduced folate carrier (RFC) protein, which also transports dihydrofolate, 5-methyl tetrahydrofolate and folinic acid [35].The gene for RFC protein is localized on chromosome 21q22, so an increased gene dosage effect as a result of chromosome 21 in DS, likely leads to entry and accumulation of higher amounts of MTX with subsequent formation of MTX polyglutamates. The increased accumulation of MTX polyglutamates in cells can be a marker of MTX toxicity [36]. Since every somatic cell in DS patients has an extra copy of chromosome 21 (constitutional trisomy), increased MTX absorption in ALLDS, especially in the GI tract, may be responsible for the severe toxicity to methotrexate observed in such patients [28, 30]. Polymorphisms in several genes concerned with folate metabolism and their association with MTX-generated toxicity have been identified. A retrospective study of 81 ALL children who had received treatment in keeping with the Dutch Childhood Oncology Group (DCOG) ALL-9 protocol, was conducted by Huang *et al*. The therapeutic regimen included high dose methotrexate (HDMTX) administration continuously as an IV infusion for a 24-hour period followed by leucovorin rescue in three doses. The results indicated that patients with *methylenetetrahydrofolate reductase (MTHFR)* 1298 AC and CC and serine *hydroxymethyl transferase (SHMT)* 1420 CT genotypes showed less toxicity to MTX, whereas *methionine synthase reductase MTRR 66* AG and GG genotypes exhibited higher toxicity [37].

A spectrum of side effects may arise from methotrexate use. Patient-to-patient variations have also been recognized. The common side effects with increased frequency and severity in DS individuals are mucositis, nausea and vomiting, diarrhoea, myelosuppression and hepatic toxicity marked by perturbations in liver enzymes (transaminases). Coagulation and pancreatic toxicities have also been reported after augmentation of methotrexate dose in post-induction phases [38]. Additionally, central nervous system (CNS) toxicity, which may precipitate in learning disabilities of a more complex and intractable nature in ALLDS than in AMLDS, has been identified [39].

An important strategy to reduce MTX toxicity is the administration of folinic acid (Leucovorin) usually between 24 and 36 hours after administering HDMTX. Leucovorin selectively rescues the normal cell from the adverse effects of methotrexate by restoring reduced folates in the normal cells so that they use it in the formation of purines and thymidine phosphate [40]. In an earlier study, Peters and Poon described methotrexate sensitivity in four patients with DS leukaemia who had received MTX in the course of treatment [41]. Severe and immediate toxic effects such as rash, diarrhoea and mucositis were detected in them irrespective mode of drug administration i.e., intravenously, intrathecally or orally. The drug became tolerable after dosing was considerably reduced (30%-50%). However, methotrexate absorption and clearance was within normal parameters in the two patients who were evaluated for it. The authors suggested the possible involvement of enzymes synthesized by genes on chromosome 21 related to purine metabolism such as tetrahydrofolate [41]. In the Medical Research Council (MRC) UKALL XI study most of the children with ALLDS did not display an unusual toxicity during the course of HDMTX therapy [42]. The authors attributed this to stringent adherence to protocols of leucovorin rescue. However, no comparison with ALLNDS children was made.

The pharmacokinetics of methotrexate in ALLDS was described by Garre *et al.* in a study designed to determine the frequency and severity of MTX toxicity in five DS ALL children, and the results were compared with NALLDS children [43]. ALLDS patients showed significantly higher toxicity in spite of having received relatively larger doses of leucovorin in anticipation of higher toxicity. Gastrointestinal toxicity was the most prominent and at high degrees (grade 2-4). Other MTX-related toxicities noted were myelosuppression up to grade 4, CNS symptoms, hepatotoxicity and maculopapular rash on skin. Repeated leucovorin in high doses may have lessened certain incidences of high toxicity to some extent but did not prevent toxic manifestations altogether. Furthermore, leucovorin reduced the occurrence and severity of mucositis, the most common feature associated with MTX toxicity, in all but one patient. In this patient, MTX doses were subsequently reduced which brought down gastrointestinal and haematological toxicities to lower grade. Drug pharmacokinetics study showed that DS patients had a greater plasma MTX concentration at 42 hours after initiating MTX therapy in comparison to ALLNDS patients which signifies altered metabolism of the drug. However, plasma MTX clearance did not materially vary between the two groups. A sevenfold risk of MTX toxicity was found to be associated with ALLDS patients. This study points to the possibility of enhanced tissue sensitivity to MTX as well as variation in drug pharmacokinetics between ALLDS and ALLNDS patients. However, a recent retrospective case controlled study of 44 ALLDS patients did not detect any clinically significant variation in the pharmacokinetics of MTX between ALLDS and ALLNDS patients. [32]. The MTX clearance rate was slower by 5% in ALLDS than in ALLNDS patients but the investigators did not deem it to be of clinical importance as, at both 24 and 48 hours, the MTX plasma concentrations between the two groups did not differ widely. As in other previous studies, this investigation also recorded a very high number of ALLDS patients displaying grade 3-4 gastrointestinal toxicity. The incidence of toxicity remained higher than that of ALLNDS patients even after dose-lowering regimens were put into effect. Patients who had received doses of mercatopurine during MTX treatment did not present with any blood related toxicity. This study [32] strongly suggests the role of differential MTX pharmacodynamics, especially in relation to the gastrointestinal mucous epithelium of the two patients groups, and highlights the possible differences in the uptake and subsequent accumulation of MTX and MTX polyglutamates (MTXPG). It seems pertinent to mention here that MTXPG remains in cells for a longer period, and increased polyglutamation could result in cellular injury and destruction of the cells of the intestinal mucosa. This may likely explain the exacerbated MTX toxic manifestations in ALLDS patients [32]. Additionally, germline polymorphisms in candidate genes may play a role in influencing the action of drug-related enzymes, proteins and drug targets, which may subsequently contribute to enhanced MTX toxicity [44]. Children with more polymorphisms have more gastrointestinal mucosa-related toxicity and hence may show altered pharmacodynamics [31].

The Ponte di Legno (PDL) study [22], the largest retrospective study to date, was conducted to explore the features of ALLDS; the data of 653 ALLDS patients who were enrolled in various international studies were analysed. It emerged that the cumulative incidence of relapse (CIR) was higher compared to that of ALLNDS patients. Moreover, the two-year period of treatment-related mortality (TRM) was higher in ALLNDS patients. These characteristics were seen to have a negative impact on the eight-year event-free survival (EFS) and overall survival (OS) of DS patients. This and several other studies compel us to further investigate the possible role of heightened MTX toxicity and its ramifications in ALLNDS individuals with regard to treatment outcomes, including TRM, EFS and OS. This remains a complex issue at best, as not only the unique constitutional patient characteristics of DS but the characteristics of leukaemic cells in the setting of DS must be considered. Additionally, interactions between MTX and other drugs that are simultaneously given to patients may complicate the issue further. Therefore, there appear to be multiple mechanisms and processes that regulate the response to this drug [19]. The literature is replete with instances where, due to toxicity-related issues, treatment protocols have been modified in which, more often than not, a reduction in MTX dose has been made. Does it affect the natural history of disease in ALLDS patients and result in poorer outcomes? The PDL study concluded that the largely dismal prognosis of ALLDS is chiefly the result of a higher rate of relapses, and TRM is a less significant factor. In light of these findings, the study does not recommend treatment reduction in general. However, for a sub-population of patients with high hyperdiploidy or *ETV6- RUNX1* mutations in which toxicity is a leading cause of death, treatment modifications including drug reduction may be opted [22].

The issue of dose reduction in ALLDS in the face of potential MTX toxicity has another aspect, i.e., an overcautious approach on the part of the treating physician leads to a reluctance to use appropriate doses of this drug. A study in DS children found that physicians used MTX and 6-mercaptopurine doses at a lesser concentration than what is prescribed in both standard protocol treatments and is also given to ALLNDS patients [45].

Significant neurological toxicity is associated with MTX use [32]. Fortunately, most of the symptoms are transient and resolve quickly, or resolve at least at the end of therapy [46]. However, there are several other studies that have investigated the long-term effects of MTX on CNS [39, 47, 48]. For ALLDS children cranial irradiation is not prescribed by any of the cancer study groups. Therefore, in such patients the effect of chemotherapy, including methotrexate therapy, on the CNS and its long-term sequelae remains a vital area for the conduction of large-scale studies. As overall survival of ALLDS patients has improved, the issue of quality of life assumes much importance. Inherently compromised brain functions unrelated to leukaemia are a feature of DS. In this setting, coupled with a higher overall toxicity to MTX, ALLDS children have a greater risk of chemotherapeutic insults to the brain with the possibility of worse long-term neuropsychological sequelae including learning disabilities and emotional problems. Intrathecal as well as intravenous MTX administration may be associated with leukoencephalopathy, cerebral cortex atrophy and seizures [48, 49]. Furthermore, an earlier study has reported that intrathecal cytosine arabinoside can augment the CNS toxicity of MTX [50]. A recent study has reported the detection of extensive vascular myelopathy of the spinal cord on an autopsy of an ALLDS patient who was given MTX therapy. The authors suggested a possible role of MTX in the processes of white matter degeneration [51]. Krull *et al.* found evidence of a direct effect of MTX on neurocognitive functions in ALL patients who were alive ten years or more after diagnosis [47]. After controlling for cranial irradiation it was determined that each 1gm/m^2 of MTX aggravated the possibility of slowed mental processing speed by 3% [47].

MTX administered in escalating doses with the initial dose of 100mg/m^2 and gradually raising it by 50mg/m^2 without following it with folinic acid rescue, until the moment toxicity is detected is also known as Capizzi MTX. This method is known to be associated with superior outcomes in standard risk ALL [38]. Larsen *et al.* in a study compared HDMTX with leucovorin rescue and Capizzi MTX in children, adolescents and young adults treated in accordance with the high-risk COG ALL protocol [52]. Better EFS was reported in the HDMTX arm than in the Capizzi MTX arm. Furthermore, fewer incidences of treatment failures including marrow and CNS failures were observed in the HDMTX arm. In the context of ALLDS patients, the mere extrapolation of these results may not be of much help to draw any clinically definitive conclusion. Clearly, there is a need to conduct clinical trials involving DS patients which could help in the way of building up a more personalized approach to treatment of DS patients. Recently, an uncommon case has been reported of a child with ALLDS who was earlier a patient of AML, who was treated successfully and remained in remission from AML when ALLDS was diagnosed at four years of age. In an intensified consolidation regimen, he was treated with an escalating dose of MTX (Capizzi MTX) given intravenously, which was not followed by leucovorin rescue. Following the second Capizzi MTX (100mg/m^2), the child developed mucositis of moderate severity and was subsequently put on a low risk maintenance regimen which had to be curtailed from three to two years. This modification fortunately had no unwanted clinical effect as the child remained disease-free until the time last reported, i.e., at seven years post-diagnosis [30].

As in the case discussed above, and in the majority of DS patients treated with MTX, mucositis emerged as the leading toxic manifestation. The intrinsically unique immunometabolism in DS coupled with the rather compromised aspect of certain components of the immune system could also be a contributory factor in mucositis. Combined with this, the effect of MTX metabolism in the setting of DS and enhancement in apoptosis of the mucosal cells breaches the cellular barriers resulting in higher grades of mucositis [30]. In a study performed to explore the metabolic and genetic components responsible for MTX toxicity, 134 childhood ALL patients were treated in line with the DCOG-ALL-10 protocol [53], and the results showed that MTX-associated mucositis was more common and frequent mainly after the first course of the drug. Besides, mucositis also accounted for the major share of overall drug related toxicity (> 3). However, since the patients had neutropenia, and, prior to starting the MTX therapy, had received drugs such as mercaptopurine, cyclophosphamide and cytarabine, the concomitant role of these drugs in aggravating the moderately severe mucositis cannot be completely ruled out [54, 55]. This might explain the higher toxicity at the end of first MTX course, since the second MTX course was not preceded by these drugs. This observation raises the possibility of interaction between drugs and their cumulative side effects, which should be further explored in every subtype of ALL including ALLDS. Since leucovorin rescue was initiated 42 hours after the commencement of the first HDMTX dose, its detoxifying effect is most likely to build up in the later phases of treatment and not in the starting phase, which also could have contributed to a higher toxicity encountered during the first course. The PDL study found that apart from reducing doses of MTX, leucovorin at a high dose was given to patients with ALLDS by the various study groups treating ALLDS patients [22]. It is plausible that a higher leucovorin dose might interfere with the efficacy of MTX by rescuing the cancer cells in addition to normal cells in ALLDS. This attenuation in the effect of MTX may have important implications for therapy and therapeutic outcomes. Several studies have shown that leucovorin in higher concentrations or its fairly early dosing after MTX administration may increase the risk of disease relapse [56, 57]. Skarby *et al.* studied the associations between disease relapse, serum methotrexate concentrations and leucovorin rescue doses in 445 children with ALL who were treated according to the Nordic Society of Pediatric Hematology and Oncology (NOPHO) ALL92 protocol [58]. Higher leucovorin doses matched with a corresponding higher MTX (which was determined by high serum MTX); the results indicated that the attempt to put into effect a heightened leucovorin rescue compromised methotrexate efficacy. Disease relapse risk was aggravated, registering a 22% increase when the leucovorin dose was doubled. This study led to the modification in the NOPHO protocol, which then prescribed a reduction in leucovorin dose. To our knowledge, no study similar to this has been conducted in ALLDS patients; however, since the ALLDS patients continue to be treated with minor modifications of the existing protocols for ALLNDS this study also holds relevance for these patients. Leucovorin doses in many instances have been intensified for ALLDS patients. Therefore, separate studies in ALLDS patients are needed to determine the impact of higher doses of leucovorin on the efficacy of HDMTX. Question remains about the optimum leucovorin dose that on the one hand would keep toxicity within tolerable limits and on the other hand would not dilute the effect of HDMTX. The enzyme dihydrofolate reductase is believed to mediate in the competitive activities of these two antagonists, i.e., MTX and leucovorin [59]. Complicating the matter is the fact that cancer patients are prescribed folate as part of a nutrient supplementation in order to increase appetite and reduce anorexia. This and the dietary folate may also influence the therapeutic effectiveness of HDMTX along with leucovorin. Studies using modern sequencing platforms may yield further information about genetic variations in enzymatic interactions and drugs that will aid in reaching a meticulous balance between MTX dose and leucovorin strength. It will also lead to a more personalized approach, the significance of which cannot be overstated in ALLDS given the heterogeneous nature of the disease [60].

The Ponte di Legno study concluded that disease relapse in ALLDS patients was the foremost cause of inferior survival. In the light of this finding it does not recommend any reduction in treatment except for a small minority genetic sub-group with *ETV6-RUNX1* or high hyperdiploidy, where toxicity-related mortality was identified to be the highest. Interestingly, this sub-group is also associated with the most favourable prognosis and a very low cumulative incidence of relapse [22]. In recent years there has been a marked improvement in EFS and OS of ALLDS children and also less disease relapse due to relatively fewer induction deaths and treatment-related mortality as compared to the pre-2000 era [61]. This is likely in part due to the emphasis laid upon not decreasing treatment intensity. Buitenkamp *et al.*, for instance have shown that usage of MTX in intermediate doses does not lead to any unexpected major toxicity issue in ALLDS children. The authors advised that 1-3g/m^2 of MTX administration coupled with meticulous observation for any unwanted toxicity should not be unsafe as a starting regimen [32]. Advances in supportive care for these patients might further improve the end results of the use of chemotherapeutic drugs including MTX.

The current treatment strategies for ALLDS patients entail a modification of treatment keeping in view the objective to limiting toxicity and minimizing treatment-related mortality. Needless to say, this is expected to have a positive impact on disease relapse as well as on the overall quality of life. In ALLDS patients the best practice is that MTX is intravenously administered in the range of 500-1000mg/m^2 with leucovorin rescue and no further augmentation of dose. The other strategy is to adopt a dose escalation regimen, starting with 500mg/m^2 and gradually escalating to 2000mg/m^2 (Capizzi MTX). In high-risk ALLDS patients, dose reductions of HDMTX should not be resorted to, and Capizzi MTX administration, where protocol dictates, should not be halted or modified in the face of apprehensions of infection. As discussed earlier, dose reductions can be made in the favourable prognosis sub-group as well as those in which minimal residual disease shows negative results [30].

5. Glucocorticoids

Glucocorticoids (GC) such as prednisolone and dexamethasone along with L-asparaginase constitute an important component of therapy for all types of ALL patients, including ALLDS patients [62]. However, usually transient hyperglycaemia has been associated with the use of glucocorticoids and L-asparaginase and studies have indicated a synergistic role of glucocorticoids and asparaginase in the development of this condition in leukaemia patients [63]. In ALLDS patients the risk of hyperglycaemia is compounded, which necessitates a more thorough observation and prompt remedial measures. In the St. Jude hospital study, Pui *et al.* showed that age, obesity and DS were each linked with a higher risk of hyperglycaemia in patients who received treatment with L-asparaginase and prednisone [64]. Additionally, in circumstances where all these traits appear together, a combinatorial effect on glucose intolerance could be witnessed. The authors also highlighted the relatively-increased blood glucose levels in hyperglycaemic DS patients as compared to non-DS patients exhibiting hyperglycaemia due to treatment [64]. Similarly, earlier studies had reported a high incidence of non-ketotic hyperosmolar diabetic coma leading to high mortality in DS children [65, 66].

It is well established that DS patients have a greater propensity to develop *diabetes mellitus,* and that too relatively earlier in life [67-69]. This has made DS an independent risk factor for a hyperglycaemic dysmetabolic state during the course of glucocorticoid therapy in ALLDS individuals [22]. A glucocorticoid-mediated hyperglycaemic dysmetabolic condition could be a contributory factor in the poor prognosis associated with ALLDS patients. Altered metabolism of glucose in ALLDS leukaemia is most likely a contributory factor that influences disease prognosis. No study in ALLDS has provided direct evidence in this regard. However, Boag *et al.* showed that non-solid tumours (pre-B ALL cells) exhibit alterations in their metabolism such as switching to exacerbated aerobic glycolysis and an increase in the number of glucose transporter GLUT 1 [70]. The authors stated that apart from tumourigenesis, the course of disease and its prognosis may also be associated with metabolic changes. A recent study has shown that dexamethasone inhibited the entry and utilization of glucose and caused disruption of glycolysis, resulting in cellular death in primary ALL blasts and ALL cell lines [71]. Furthermore, higher apoptosis was identified in those cells in which glucose concentration was relatively low, which reveals that an efficient and higher apoptotic rate could be reached under lower glycaemic conditions. These studies should be reproduced in ALLDS individuals and results thus obtained would help better address the issue of hyperglycaemia in ALLDS as altered metabolism is generally more common in DS [17, 28, 30], also, in the light of the findings that glucocorticoid sensitivity could play a critical role in influencing treatment outcomes and the increased resistance to these hormones could lead to a worsening prognosis. Holleman and colleagues have described that genes related to glucose metabolism are highly expressed in the cells resistant to glucocorticoids [72]. Notably this was detected in patients with pre-B ALL cells, and the overwhelming majority of ALLDS belongs to the pre-B cell phenotype [18]. Moreover, enhanced glycolysis in cells exacerbates the risk for glucocorticoid resistance in leukaemic lymphoblasts [73]. Identification and targeting of the upregulated genes and the genetic pathways involved in the generation of higher glycolysis in DS patients in future may prove to be advantageous.

Prednisolone and dexamethasone have both been in use in ALL for decades, especially in the remission induction phase of therapy. However, studies have indicated better treatment results with the use of dexamethasone, especially in the context of the higher efficacy of dexamethasone in penetrating the blood brain barrier, leading to a lower rate of CNS relapse [74-77] and meningeal leukaemia [78]. However, dexamethasone use is associated with a higher drug toxicity and a higher rate of infections. Higher infections, partly as a result of therapy causing myelosuppression, is well known in DS patients. Recently, Domenech *et al.*

have shown that dexamethasone at 6mg/m^2/day and prednisolone at 60mg/m^2/day exert equal benefits and that no significant variation in toxicities have been detected in the use of these two drugs at the tested dosing [79]. However, the majority opinion seems to be that dexamethasone is a better choice as far as improved CNS control is concerned. Enhanced steroid toxicity could also manifest as myopathy and a marked increase in weight. DS individuals independently show a predilection towards more weight gain [17]. Which of the two drugs, dexamethasone or prednisolone, can lead to greater weight gain or exert an equal effect is a moot question. Genetic profiling of patients in the context of glucocorticoid activities combined with metabolomic studies may give some direction in the future. Very recently, Bindreither *et al.* studied the transcriptional profile of T-ALL cells after treating them with prednisolone and dexamethasone, which showed no remarkable variations in the transcriptional responses detected [80]. These results also highlight that both of these glucocorticoids regulated identical genes. Furthermore, the authors conclude that the differential treatment outcomes of dexamethasone and prednisolone, as reported in several studies, are perhaps due to differences in the pharmacokinetics and pharmacodynamics of these drugs. Studies dissecting the metabolic and molecular pathways involved in the glucocorticoid response in DS patients will help to inform practitioners to adjust and improve therapy. As of now, the point made by Inaba and Pui holds relevance that, in view of the fact that considerable variations are encountered among patients with regard to the sensitivity of ALL cells, and the same for glucocorticoid toxicity, best practice would be to consider the risk of relapse, phase of therapy and the drugs that are administered concomitantly with the glucocorticoids, before opting for a particular glucocorticoid [62]. Currently, in delayed intensification therapy for ALLDS patients, MRC UK and COG cancer groups recommend discontinuous dexamethasone dosing [18, 30].

6. Anthracyclines and Cytarabine (Ara –C)

Anthracyclines, mainly daunorubicin, doxorubicin and idarubicin, are used in the therapeutic regimens for treating ALL as well as AML [15, 81]. These anti-tumour antibiotics bind to DNA and prevent the unwinding activity of topoisomerase, which leads to abrogation of the process of DNA replication. Cytarabine (ara-C) incorporates into DNA through its active metabolite and impedes the binding of d-CTP to DNA. It abrogates the activity of the DNA polymerase enzyme [28]. In current treatment strategies, ara-C has taken the central stage for AML treatment, including AMLDS.

In ALLDS patients, anthracycline use is advocated differently by the groups. The Dutch Children Oncology Group (DCOG) and France Acute Lymphoblastic Leukaemia (FRALLE) do not use anthracyclines for induction therapy at all, whereas, daunorubicin induction is given by some groups in the case of patients with inadequate response. Anthracycline, along with glucocorticoids were given in the induction phase by physicians at St. Jude Research Hospital, fortunately with no reported unexpected toxicities. For further improvement in survival and lowering toxicities especially cardiac toxicity, further trials and research studies are greatly needed so that the optimum balance of modern therapy can be reached in the different risk groups of patients with ALLDS [18].

Several studies have been conducted in AMLDS patients to determine the effects, side effects and efficacy of anthracycline, which also highlights the altered drug response and unique genetic and metabolic make up of AMLDS individuals. Unlike ALLDS, AMLDS children have a better outcome with the highest curative rate of any other group of myeloid leukaemia patients [16, 82, 83]. The French American British Classification (FAB) classification AML M7 is characterized by one of the worst prognoses in children without DS. However, the situation is different in the context of acute megakaryoblastic leukaemia (AMkL) DS, especially in children younger than three years of age, where excellent prognosis in recent years has generally been acknowledged [18, 84]. AMkL happens to be the most common phenotype in AMLDS [19].

Increased sensitivity to anthracycline and other drugs can be attributed to the presence of a high level of oxygen free radicals which are inherent in the cellular constituents of DS individuals [28, 85]. The enhanced ROS production coupled with perturbation in superoxide dismutase observed in DS, in the absence of concomitant increase in other antioxidant enzymes such as catalase and glutathione peroxidase, predisposes the cells to undergo apoptosis. In this altered metabolic state, drug-induced apoptosis is further exaggerated. It has been proposed that the HAS 21-linked gene dosage effect of NADH dehydrogenase ubiquinone flavoproein 3 may be responsible for increased ROS production through enhanced mitochondrial respiration [84]. Reduced anthracycline dosage is now universally prescribed for AMLDS patients, especially to obviate the well-known cardiotoxicity associated with anthracycline therapy. This is particularly beneficial to DS individuals as they are prone to mitochondrial dysfunction and thereby increased cardiac oxidative stress [86].

The well-known favourable prognosis in AMLDS children reflects the enhanced sensitivity of leukaemic blasts to cytarabine (ara-C) and anthracyclines [87-89]. The modification of cancer drug metabolism including ara-C in AMLDS individuals has been the subject of extensive research. A landmark study by Taub *et al.* found that DS myeloblasts showed an enhanced sensitivity to ara-C, which was ascribed as being a contributory factor to better prognosis. This is further supported by the observations that both DS myeloblasts as well as trisomy 21 lymphoblastoid cell lines accumulate higher ara-CTP (a metabolite of ara-C synthesis) levels than non-DS cells. Taken together, these observations imply an altered metabolism of ara-C in DS children. However, other factors like the concomitant use of daunorubicin or the gene dosage effect of enzymes related to chromosome 21 such as carbonyl reductase and superoxide dismutase (SOD) may also influence outcomes in AMLDS patients [16]. Zwaan *et al.* showed that AMLDS cells were 12 times more sensitive to ara-C than AMLNDS cells [89]. The authors also determined a two- to seven-fold heightened anthracycline sensitivity in AMLDS cells. In another study, AMLDS cells showed a several-fold increase in sensitivity to both ara-C and daunorubicin in MTT drug assays. Besides, a remarkably higher concentration of ara-CTP was also detected, which strongly pointed to a link between trisomy 21 and high drug sensitivity [90]. Other studies have strengthened this view and implicate an altered metabolism of both ara–C and daunorubicin in AMLDS children [88, 89].

Mutations in the GATA1 transcription factor gene present on chromosome X is an exclusive feature of AMkLDS [29]. These mutations likely contribute to augmented ara-C sensitivity. GATA1 mutants were found to have a truncated 40 KDa protein in AMLDS blasts instead of the wild-type 50 KDa protein [29]. This affects cytidine deaminase (CDA) gene expression, which is believed to result in less CDA expression in DS myeloid blasts, accounting for the increased ara-C sensitivity. Another factor that might play a role in increased ara-C sensitivity is the alteration in folate metabolism, which is traced to the heightened activity of the CBS enzyme linked to HSA21.

7. Future directions in pharmacotherapy

With an increased longevity of DS individuals, new challenges have arisen in the area of the management and treatment of associated morbidities. An increasing age carries the potential to modify the natural history of the disease. Additionally, in DS the phenomenon of accelerated ageing, and thereby accompanied changes in metabolism, is a factor that can hardly be ignored. A better understanding of drug metabolism in DS is extremely useful because DS individuals receive several medicines as part of their palliative care and to combat concomitant illnesses. Further collaborative studies in a larger DS cohort are warranted to better understand the phenomenon of altered drug metabolism and concomitant drug interactions. DS is characterized by phenotypic heterogeneity, and the varying severity and complexity of the disease involves multi-organ systems. Given the wide spectrum of clinical anomalies in DS, future pharmacotherapy approaches need a more tailored approach for personalized medicine based on advanced knowledge and input from drug metabolism studies in DS individuals. Thus, further research and information from case studies and drug trials are warranted to adopt appropriate treatment regimes. It may also be relevant to neurodegenerative diseases such as dementia and Alzheimer's, which have an earlier onset in DS and are also prevalent in a large proportion of elderly people in the general population.

Author details

Jumana Y. Alaama[1*], Muhammad S. Ahmad[2], Sultan Ahmad[2] and Zoheir A. Damanhouri[3]

*Address all correspondence to: jalama@kau.edu.sa

1 Department of Medical Genetics, Faculty of Medicine, Princess Al-Jawhara AlBrahim Center of Excellence in Research of Hereditary Disorders, King Abdulaziz University, Jeddah, Saudi Arabia

2 King Fahd Medical Research Center, King Abdulaziz University, Jeddah, Saudi Arabia

3 Department of Pharmacology, Faculty of Medicine, King Abdulaziz University, Jeddah, Saudi Arabia

References

[1] S. E. Parker, C. T. Mai, M. A. Canfield, R. Rickard, Y. Wang, R. E. Meyer, P. Anderson, C. A. Mason, J. S. Collins, R. S. Kirby, and A. Correa, 'Updated National Birth Prevalence estimates for selected birth defects in the United States, 2004-2006', *Birth Defects Res. A. Clin. Mol. Teratol.*, vol. 88, no. 12, pp. 1008–16, Dec. 2010.

[2] K. Kim, Y. Wang, R. S. Kirby, and C. M. Druschel, 'Prevalence and trends of selected congenital malformations in New York State, 1983 to 2007', *Birth Defects Res. A. Clin. Mol. Teratol.*, vol. 97, no. 10, pp. 619–27, Oct. 2013.

[3] J. E. Kucik, M. Shin, C. Siffel, L. Marengo, and A. Correa, 'Trends in survival among children with Down syndrome in 10 regions of the United States', *Pediatrics*, vol. 131, no. 1, pp. 27–36, Jan. 2013.

[4] M. Shin, L. M. Besser, J. E. Kucik, C. Lu, C. Siffel, and A. Correa, 'Prevalence of Down syndrome among children and adolescents in 10 regions of the United States', *Pediatrics*, vol. 124, no. 6, pp. 1565–71, Dec. 2009.

[5] M. Hattori, A. Fujiyama, T. D. Taylor, H. Watanabe, T. Yada, H. S. Park, A. Toyoda, K. Ishii, Y. Totoki, D. K. Choi, Y. Groner, E. Soeda, M. Ohki, T. Takagi, Y. Sakaki, S. Taudien, K. Blechschmidt, A. Polley, U. Menzel, J. Delabar, K. Kumpf, R. Lehmann, D. Patterson, K. Reichwald, A. Rump, M. Schillhabel, A. Schudy, W. Zimmermann, A. Rosenthal, J. Kudoh, K. Schibuya, K. Kawasaki, S. Asakawa, A. Shintani, T. Sasaki, K. Nagamine, S. Mitsuyama, S. E. Antonarakis, S. Minoshima, N. Shimizu, G. Nordsiek, K. Hornischer, P. Brant, M. Scharfe, O. Schon, A. Desario, J. Reichelt, G. Kauer, H. Blocker, J. Ramser, A. Beck, S. Klages, S. Hennig, L. Riesselmann, E. Dagand, T. Haaf, S. Wehrmeyer, K. Borzym, K. Gardiner, D. Nizetic, F. Francis, H. Lehrach, R. Reinhardt, and M. L. Yaspo, 'The DNA sequence of human chromosome 21', *Nature*, vol. 405, no. 6784, pp. 311–9, May 2000.

[6] D. Patterson, 'Molecular genetic analysis of Down syndrome', *Hum. Genet.*, vol. 126, no. 1, pp. 195–214, Jul. 2009.

[7] P. Varga, A. V Oláh, and E. Oláh, '[Biochemical alterations in patients with Down syndrome]', *Orv. Hetil.*, vol. 149, no. 26, pp. 1203–13, Jun. 2008.

[8] K. Uyeda, 'Phosphofructokinase', *Adv. Enzymol. Relat. Areas Mol. Biol.*, vol. 48, pp. 193–244, Jan. 1979.

[9] S. Vora and U. Francke, 'Assignment of the human gene for liver-type 6-phosphofructokinase isozyme (PFKL) to chromosome 21 by using somatic cell hybrids and monoclonal anti-L antibody', *Proc. Natl. Acad. Sci. U. S. A.*, vol. 78, no. 6, pp. 3738–42, Jun. 1981.

[10] H. Nakajima, '[Phosphofructokinase (PFK)]', *Nihon Rinsho.*, vol. 53, no. 5, pp. 1241–6, May 1995.

[11] M. Peled-Kamar, H. Degani, P. Bendel, R. Margalit, and Y. Groner, 'Altered brain glucose metabolism in transgenic-PFKL mice with elevated L-phosphofructokinase: in vivo NMR studies', *Brain Res.*, vol. 810, no. 1–2, pp. 138–45, Nov. 1998.

[12] A. Elson, D. Levanon, Y. Weiss, and Y. Groner, 'Overexpression of liver-type phosphofructokinase (PFKL) in transgenic-PFKL mice: implication for gene dosage in trisomy 21', *Biochem. J.*, vol. 299 Pt 2, pp. 409–15, Apr. 1994.

[13] M. S. Ebadi and R. B. Kugel, 'Alteration in metabolism of acetylsalicylic acid in children with Down's syndrome: decreased plasma binding and formation of Salicyluric Acid', *Pediatr. Res.*, vol. 4, no. 2, pp. 187–93, Mar. 1970.

[14] H. Hasle, I. H. Clemmensen, and M. Mikkelsen, 'Risks of leukaemia and solid tumours in individuals with Down's syndrome', *Lancet*, vol. 355, no. 9199, pp. 165–9, Jan. 2000.

[15] K. R. Rabin and J. A. Whitlock, 'Malignancy in children with trisomy 21', *Oncologist*, vol. 14, no. 2, pp. 164–73, Feb. 2009.

[16] J. W. Taub, L. H. Matherly, M. L. Stout, S. A. Buck, J. G. Gurney, and Y. Ravindranath, 'Enhanced metabolism of 1-beta-D-arabinofuranosylcytosine in Down syndrome cells: a contributing factor to the superior event free survival of Down syndrome children with acute myeloid leukemia', *Blood*, vol. 87, no. 8, pp. 3395–403, Apr. 1996.

[17] N. J. Roizen and D. Patterson, 'Down's syndrome', *Lancet*, vol. 361, no. 9365, pp. 1281–9, May 2003.

[18] K. W. Maloney, J. W. Taub, Y. Ravindranath, I. Roberts, and P. Vyas, 'Down syndrome preleukemia and leukemia', *Pediatr. Clin. North Am.*, vol. 62, no. 1, pp. 121–37, Feb. 2015.

[19] A. C. Xavier and J. W. Taub, 'Acute leukemia in children with Down syndrome', *Haematologica*, vol. 95, no. 7, pp. 1043–5, Jul. 2010.

[20] L. Hertzberg, E. Vendramini, I. Ganmore, G. Cazzaniga, M. Schmitz, J. Chalker, R. Shiloh, I. Iacobucci, C. Shochat, S. Zeligson, G. Cario, M. Stanulla, S. Strehl, L. J. Russell, C. J. Harrison, B. Bornhauser, A. Yoda, G. Rechavi, D. Bercovich, A. Borkhardt, H. Kempski, G. te Kronnie, J.-P. Bourquin, E. Domany, and S. Izraeli, 'Down syndrome acute lymphoblastic leukemia, a highly heterogeneous disease in which aberrant expression of CRLF2 is associated with mutated JAK2: a report from the International BFM Study Group', *Blood*, vol. 115, no. 5, pp. 1006–17, Feb. 2010.

[21] D. Grimwade and S. D. Freeman, 'Defining minimal residual disease in acute myeloid leukemia: which platforms are ready for "prime time"?', *Blood*, vol. 124, no. 23, pp. 3345–55, Nov. 2014.

[22] T. D. Buitenkamp, S. Izraeli, M. Zimmermann, E. Forestier, N. A. Heerema, M. M. van den Heuvel-Eibrink, R. Pieters, C. M. Korbijn, L. B. Silverman, K. Schmiegelow,

D.-C. Liang, K. Horibe, M. Arico, A. Biondi, G. Basso, K. R. Rabin, M. Schrappe, G. Cario, G. Mann, M. Morak, R. Panzer-Grümayer, V. Mondelaers, T. Lammens, H. Cavé, B. Stark, I. Ganmore, A. V Moorman, A. Vora, S. P. Hunger, C.-H. Pui, C. G. Mullighan, A. Manabe, G. Escherich, J. R. Kowalczyk, J. A. Whitlock, and C. M. Zwaan, 'Acute lymphoblastic leukemia in children with Down syndrome: a retrospective analysis from the Ponte di Legno study group', *Blood*, vol. 123, no. 1, pp. 70–7, Jan. 2014.

[23] Y. Ravindranath, 'Recent advances in pediatric acute lymphoblastic and myeloid leukemia', *Curr. Opin. Oncol.*, vol. 15, no. 1, pp. 23–35, Jan. 2003.

[24] K. W. Maloney, 'Acute lymphoblastic leukaemia in children with Down syndrome: an updated review', *Br. J. Haematol.*, vol. 155, no. 4, pp. 420–5, Nov. 2011.

[25] A. D. Sorrell, T. A. Alonzo, J. M. Hilden, R. B. Gerbing, T. W. Loew, L. Hathaway, D. Barnard, J. W. Taub, Y. Ravindranath, F. O. Smith, R. J. Arceci, W. G. Woods, and A. S. Gamis, 'Favorable survival maintained in children who have myeloid leukemia associated with Down syndrome using reduced-dose chemotherapy on Children's Oncology Group trial A2971: a report from the Children's Oncology Group', *Cancer*, vol. 118, no. 19, pp. 4806–14, Oct. 2012.

[26] C.-H. Pui and W. E. Evans, 'Treatment of acute lymphoblastic leukemia', *N. Engl. J. Med.*, vol. 354, no. 2, pp. 166–78, Jan. 2006.

[27] L. Wang, H. L. McLeod, and R. M. Weinshilboum, 'Genomics and drug response', *N. Engl. J. Med.*, vol. 364, no. 12, pp. 1144–53, Mar. 2011.

[28] J. W. Taub and Y. Ge, 'Down syndrome, drug metabolism and chromosome 21', *Pediatr. Blood Cancer*, vol. 44, no. 1, pp. 33–9, Jan. 2005.

[29] Y. Ge, T. L. Jensen, M. L. Stout, R. M. Flatley, P. J. Grohar, Y. Ravindranath, L. H. Matherly, and J. W. Taub, 'The role of cytidine deaminase and GATA1 mutations in the increased cytosine arabinoside sensitivity of Down syndrome myeloblasts and leukemia cell lines', *Cancer Res.*, vol. 64, no. 2, pp. 728–35, Jan. 2004.

[30] S. Izraeli, A. Vora, C. M. Zwaan, and J. Whitlock, 'How I treat ALL in Down's syndrome: pathobiology and management', *Blood*, vol. 123, no. 1, pp. 35–40, Jan. 2014.

[31] S. Kishi, C. Cheng, D. French, D. Pei, S. Das, E. H. Cook, N. Hijiya, C. Rizzari, G. L. Rosner, T. Frudakis, C.-H. Pui, W. E. Evans, and M. V Relling, 'Ancestry and pharmacogenetics of antileukemic drug toxicity', *Blood*, vol. 109, no. 10, pp. 4151–7, May 2007.

[32] T. D. Buitenkamp, R. A. A. Mathôt, V. de Haas, R. Pieters, and C. M. Zwaan, 'Methotrexate-induced side effects are not due to differences in pharmacokinetics in children with Down syndrome and acute lymphoblastic leukemia', *Haematologica*, vol. 95, no. 7, pp. 1106–13, Jul. 2010.

[33] E. S. L. Chan and B. N. Cronstein, 'Mechanisms of action of methotrexate', *Bull. Hosp. Jt. Dis.*, vol. 71 Suppl 1, pp. S5–8, Jan. 2013.

[34] S. P. Treon and B. A. Chabner, 'Concepts in use of high-dose methotrexate therapy', *Clin. Chem.*, vol. 42, no. 8 Pt 2, pp. 1322–9, Aug. 1996.

[35] P. De Marco, M. G. Calevo, A. Moroni, E. Merello, A. Raso, R. H. Finnell, H. Zhu, L. Andreussi, A. Cama, and V. Capra, 'Reduced folate carrier polymorphism (80A-->G) and neural tube defects', *Eur. J. Hum. Genet.*, vol. 11, no. 3, pp. 245–52, Mar. 2003.

[36] L. Kager, M. Cheok, W. Yang, G. Zaza, Q. Cheng, J. C. Panetta, C.-H. Pui, J. R. Downing, M. V Relling, and W. E. Evans, 'Folate pathway gene expression differs in subtypes of acute lymphoblastic leukemia and influences methotrexate pharmacodynamics', *J. Clin. Invest.*, vol. 115, no. 1, pp. 110–7, Jan. 2005.

[37] L. Huang, W. J. E. Tissing, R. de Jonge, B. D. van Zelst, and R. Pieters, 'Polymorphisms in folate-related genes: association with side effects of high-dose methotrexate in childhood acute lymphoblastic leukemia', *Leukemia*, vol. 22, no. 9, pp. 1798–800, Sep. 2008.

[38] Y. Matloub, B. C. Bostrom, S. P. Hunger, L. C. Stork, A. Angiolillo, H. Sather, M. La, J. M. Gastier-Foster, N. A. Heerema, S. Sailer, P. J. Buckley, B. Thomson, C. Cole, J. B. Nachman, G. Reaman, N. Winick, W. L. Carroll, M. Devidas, and P. S. Gaynon, 'Escalating intravenous methotrexate improves event-free survival in children with standard-risk acute lymphoblastic leukemia: a report from the Children's Oncology Group', *Blood*, vol. 118, no. 2, pp. 243–51, Jul. 2011.

[39] C. Roncadin, J. Hitzler, A. Downie, I. Montour-Proulx, C. Alyman, E. Cairney, and B. J. Spiegler, 'Neuropsychological late effects of treatment for acute leukemia in children with down syndrome', *Pediatr. Blood Cancer*, vol. 62, no. 5, pp. 854–8, Dec. 2014

[40] S. P. Ackland and R. L. Schilsky, 'High-dose methotrexate: a critical reappraisal', *J. Clin. Oncol.*, vol. 5, no. 12, pp. 2017–31, Dec. 1987.

[41] M. Peeters and A. Poon, 'Down syndrome and leukemia: unusual clinical aspects and unexpected methotrexate sensitivity', *Eur. J. Pediatr.*, vol. 146, no. 4, pp. 416–22, Jul. 1987.

[42] J. M. Chessells, G. Harrison, S. M. Richards, C. C. Bailey, F. G. Hill, B. E. Gibson, and I. M. Hann, 'Down's syndrome and acute lymphoblastic leukaemia: clinical features and response to treatment', *Arch. Dis. Child.*, vol. 85, no. 4, pp. 321–5, Oct. 2001.

[43] M. L. Garré, M. V Relling, D. Kalwinsky, R. Dodge, W. R. Crom, M. Abromowitch, C. H. Pui, and W. E. Evans, 'Pharmacokinetics and toxicity of methotrexate in children with Down syndrome and acute lymphocytic leukemia', *J. Pediatr.*, vol. 111, no. 4, pp. 606–12, Oct. 1987.

[44] M. H. Cheok and W. E. Evans, 'Acute lymphoblastic leukaemia: a model for the pharmacogenomics of cancer therapy', *Nat. Rev. Cancer*, vol. 6, no. 2, pp. 117–29, Feb. 2006.

[45] C. Bohnstedt, M. Levinsen, S. Rosthøj, B. Zeller, M. Taskinen, S. Hafsteinsdottir, H. Björgvinsdóttir, M. Heyman, and K. Schmiegelow, 'Physicians compliance during maintenance therapy in children with Down syndrome and acute lymphoblastic leukemia', *Leukemia*, vol. 27, no. 4, pp. 866–70, Apr. 2013.

[46] D. Bhojwani, N. D. Sabin, D. Pei, J. J. Yang, R. B. Khan, J. C. Panetta, K. R. Krull, H. Inaba, J. E. Rubnitz, M. L. Metzger, S. C. Howard, R. C. Ribeiro, C. Cheng, W. E. Reddick, S. Jeha, J. T. Sandlund, W. E. Evans, C.-H. Pui, and M. V Relling, 'Methotrexate-induced neurotoxicity and leukoencephalopathy in childhood acute lymphoblastic leukemia', *J. Clin. Oncol.*, vol. 32, no. 9, pp. 949–59, Mar. 2014.

[47] K. R. Krull, T. M. Brinkman, C. Li, G. T. Armstrong, K. K. Ness, D. K. Srivastava, J. G. Gurney, C. Kimberg, M. J. Krasin, C.-H. Pui, L. L. Robison, and M. M. Hudson, 'Neurocognitive outcomes decades after treatment for childhood acute lymphoblastic leukemia: a report from the St Jude lifetime cohort study', *J. Clin. Oncol.*, vol. 31, no. 35, pp. 4407–15, Dec. 2013.

[48] C. C. Peterson, C. E. Johnson, L. Y. Ramirez, S. Huestis, A. L. H. Pai, H. A. Demaree, and D. Drotar, 'A meta-analysis of the neuropsychological sequelae of chemotherapy-only treatment for pediatric acute lymphoblastic leukemia', *Pediatr. Blood Cancer*, vol. 51, no. 1, pp. 99–104, Jul. 2008.

[49] M. Moleski, 'Neuropsychological, neuroanatomical, and neurophysiological consequences of CNS chemotherapy for acute lymphoblastic leukemia', *Arch. Clin. Neuropsychol.*, vol. 15, no. 7, pp. 603–30, Oct. 2000.

[50] J. Giralt, J. J. Ortega, T. Olive, R. Verges, I. Forio, and L. Salvador, 'Long-term neuropsychologic sequelae of childhood leukemia: comparison of two CNS prophylactic regimens', *Int. J. Radiat. Oncol. Biol. Phys.*, vol. 24, no. 1, pp. 49–53, Jan. 1992.

[51] K. Satomi, M. Yoshida, K. Matsuoka, H. Okita, Y. Hosoya, Y. Shioda, M.-A. Kumagai, T. Mori, Y. Morishita, M. Noguchi, and A. Nakazawa, 'Myelopathy mimicking subacute combined degeneration in a Down syndrome patient with methotrexate treatment for B lymphoblastic leukemia: report of an autopsy case', *Neuropathology*, vol. 34, no. 4, pp. 414–9, Aug. 2014.

[52] E. C. Larsen, W. L. Salzer, M. Devidas, J. B. Nachman, E. A. Raetz, M. L. Loh, N. A. Heerema, A. J. Carroll, J. M. Gastier-Foster, M. J. Borowitz, B. L. Wood, C. L. Willman, N. J. Winick, S. Hunger, and W. L. Carroll, 'Comparison of high-dose methotrexate (HD-MTX) with Capizzi methotrexate plus asparaginase (C-MTX/ASNase) in children and young adults with high-risk acute lymphoblastic leukemia (HR-ALL): A report from the Children's Oncology Group Study AALL0232', *ASCO Meet. Abstr.*, vol. 29, no. 18_suppl, p. 3, Jun. 2011.

[53] M. A. H. den Hoed, E. Lopez-Lopez, M. L. Te Winkel, W. Tissing, J. D. E. de Rooij, A. Gutierrez-Camino, A. Garcia-Orad, E. den Boer, R. Pieters, S. M. F. Pluijm, R. de Jonge, and M. M. van den Heuvel-Eibrink, 'Genetic and metabolic determinants of methotrexate-induced mucositis in pediatric acute lymphoblastic leukemia', *Pharmacogenomics J.*, Nov. 2014.

[54] P. B. van Kooten Niekerk, K. Schmiegelow, and H. Schroeder, 'Influence of methylene tetrahydrofolate reductase polymorphisms and coadministration of antimetabolites on toxicity after high dose methotrexate', *Eur. J. Haematol.*, vol. 81, no. 5, pp. 391–8, Nov. 2008.

[55] P. Niscola, C. Romani, L. Cupelli, L. Scaramucci, A. Tendas, T. Dentamaro, S. Amadori, and P. de Fabritiis, 'Mucositis in patients with hematologic malignancies: an overview', *Haematologica*, vol. 92, no. 2, pp. 222–31, Feb. 2007.

[56] N. Graf, W. Jost, J. Müller, H. E. Keller, and F. C. Sitzmann, 'The effect of methotrexate pharmacokinetics and of leucovorin rescue on the prognosis of osteosarcoma', *Klin. Pädiatrie*, vol. 202, no. 5, pp. 340–6, Jan. 1990.

[57] J. Sterba, L. Dusek, R. Demlova, and D. Valik, 'Pretreatment plasma folate modulates the pharmacodynamic effect of high-dose methotrexate in children with acute lymphoblastic leukemia and non-Hodgkin lymphoma: 'folate overrescue' concept revisited', *Clin. Chem.*, vol. 52, no. 4, pp. 692–700, Apr. 2006.

[58] T. V. C. Skärby, H. Anderson, J. Heldrup, J. A. Kanerva, H. Seidel, and K. Schmiegelow, 'High leucovorin doses during high-dose methotrexate treatment may reduce the cure rate in childhood acute lymphoblastic leukemia', *Leukemia*, vol. 20, no. 11, pp. 1955–62, Nov. 2006.

[59] D. M. Boarman, J. Baram, and C. J. Allegra, 'Mechanism of leucovorin reversal of methotrexate cytotoxicity in human MCF-7 breast cancer cells', *Biochem. Pharmacol.*, vol. 40, no. 12, pp. 2651–60, Dec. 1990.

[60] K. Robien, 'Folate during antifolate chemotherapy: what we know... and do not know' *Nutr. Clin. Pract.*, vol. 20, no. 4, pp. 411–22, Aug. 2005.

[61] F. Meyr, G. Escherich, G. Mann, T. Klingebiel, A. Kulozik, C. Rossig, M. Schrappe, G. Henze, A. von Stackelberg, and J. Hitzler, 'Outcomes of treatment for relapsed acute lymphoblastic leukaemia in children with Down syndrome', *Br. J. Haematol.*, vol. 162, no. 1, pp. 98–106, Jul. 2013.

[62] H. Inaba and C.-H. Pui, 'Glucocorticoid use in acute lymphoblastic leukaemia', *Lancet. Oncol.*, vol. 11, no. 11, pp. 1096–106, Nov. 2010.

[63] A. M. Spinola-Castro, A. A. Siviero-Miachon, S. Andreoni, P. D. C. Tosta-Hernandez, C. R. P. D. Macedo, and M. L. de M. Lee, 'Transient hyperglycemia during childhood acute lymphocytic leukemia chemotherapy: an old event revisited', *Clin. Adv. Hematol. Oncol.*, vol. 7, no. 7, pp. 465–72, Jul. 2009.

[64] C. H. Pui, G. A. Burghen, W. P. Bowman, and R. J. Aur, 'Risk factors for hyperglycemia in children with leukemia receiving L-asparaginase and prednisone', *J. Pediatr.*, vol. 99, no. 1, pp. 46–50, Jul. 1981.

[65] H. M. Rubin, R. Kramer, and A. Drash, 'Hyperosmolality complicating diabetes mellitus in childhood', *J. Pediatr.*, vol. 74, no. 2, pp. 177–86, Feb. 1969.

[66] M. M. Belmonte, E. Colle, D. A. Murphy, and F. W. Wiglesworth, 'Nonketotic hyperosmolar diabetic coma in Down's syndrome', *J. Pediatr.*, vol. 77, no. 5, pp. 879–81, Nov. 1970.

[67] M. Bassal, M. K. La, J. A. Whitlock, H. N. Sather, N. A. Heerema, P. S. Gaynon, and L. C. Stork, 'Lymphoblast biology and outcome among children with Down syndrome and ALL treated on CCG-1952', *Pediatr. Blood Cancer*, vol. 44, no. 1, pp. 21–8, Jan. 2005.

[68] A. Milunsky and P. W. Neurath, 'Diabetes mellitus in Down's Syndrome', *Arch. Environ. Health*, vol. 17, no. 3, pp. 372–6, Sep. 1968.

[69] A. J. Anwar, J. D. Walker, and B. M. Frier, 'Type 1 diabetes mellitus and Down's syndrome: prevalence, management and diabetic complications', *Diabet. Med.*, vol. 15, no. 2, pp. 160–3, Feb. 1998.

[70] J. M. Boag, A. H. Beesley, M. J. Firth, J. R. Freitas, J. Ford, K. Hoffmann, A. J. Cummings, N. H. de Klerk, and U. R. Kees, 'Altered glucose metabolism in childhood pre-B acute lymphoblastic leukaemia', *Leukemia*, vol. 20, no. 10, pp. 1731–7, Oct. 2006.

[71] E. Buentke, A. Nordström, H. Lin, A.-C. Björklund, E. Laane, M. Harada, L. Lu, T. Tegnebratt, S. Stone-Elander, M. Heyman, S. Söderhäll, A. Porwit, C.-G. Ostenson, M. Shoshan, K. P. Tamm, and D. Grandér, 'Glucocorticoid-induced cell death is mediated through reduced glucose metabolism in lymphoid leukemia cells', *Blood Cancer J.*, vol. 1, no. 7, p. e31, Jul. 2011.

[72] A. Holleman, M. H. Cheok, M. L. den Boer, W. Yang, A. J. P. Veerman, K. M. Kazemier, D. Pei, C. Cheng, C.-H. Pui, M. V Relling, G. E. Janka-Schaub, R. Pieters, and W. E. Evans, 'Gene-expression patterns in drug-resistant acute lymphoblastic leukemia cells and response to treatment', *N. Engl. J. Med.*, vol. 351, no. 6, pp. 533–42, Aug. 2004.

[73] E. Hulleman, K. M. Kazemier, A. Holleman, D. J. VanderWeele, C. M. Rudin, M. J. C. Broekhuis, W. E. Evans, R. Pieters, and M. L. Den Boer, 'Inhibition of glycolysis modulates prednisolone resistance in acute lymphoblastic leukemia cells', *Blood*, vol. 113, no. 9, pp. 2014–21, Feb. 2009.

[74] J. F. Holland and O. Glidewell, 'Chemotherapy of acute lymphocytic leukemia of childhood', *Cancer*, vol. 30, no. 6, pp. 1480–7, Dec. 1972.

[75] C. D. Mitchell, S. M. Richards, S. E. Kinsey, J. Lilleyman, A. Vora, and T. O. B. Eden, 'Benefit of dexamethasone compared with prednisolone for childhood acute lympho-

blastic leukaemia: results of the UK Medical Research Council ALL97 randomized trial', *Br. J. Haematol.*, vol. 129, no. 6, pp. 734–45, Jun. 2005.

[76] F. M. Balis, C. M. Lester, G. P. Chrousos, R. L. Heideman, and D. G. Poplack, 'Differences in cerebrospinal fluid penetration of corticosteroids: possible relationship to the prevention of meningeal leukemia', *J. Clin. Oncol.*, vol. 5, no. 2, pp. 202–7, Feb. 1987.

[77] C.-H. Pui, C. G. Mullighan, W. E. Evans, and M. V Relling, 'Pediatric acute lymphoblastic leukemia: where are we going and how do we get there?', *Blood*, vol. 120, no. 6, pp. 1165–74, Aug. 2012.

[78] B. Jones, A. I. Freeman, J. J. Shuster, C. Jacquillat, M. Weil, C. Pochedly, L. Sinks, L. Chevalier, H. M. Maurer, and K. Koch, 'Lower incidence of meningeal leukemia when prednisone is replaced by dexamethasone in the treatment of acute lymphocytic leukemia', *Med. Pediatr. Oncol.*, vol. 19, no. 4, pp. 269–75, Jan. 1991.

[79] C. Domenech, S. Suciu, B. De Moerloose, F. Mazingue, G. Plat, A. Ferster, A. Uyttebroeck, N. Sirvent, P. Lutz, K. Yakouben, M. Munzer, P. Röhrlich, D. Plantaz, F. Millot, P. Philippet, N. Dastugue, S. Girard, H. Cavé, Y. Benoit, and Y. Bertrandfor, 'Dexamethasone (6 mg/m^2/day) and prednisolone (60 mg/m^2/day) were equally effective as induction therapy for childhood acute lymphoblastic leukemia in the EORTC CLG 58951 randomized trial', *Haematologica*, vol. 99, no. 7, pp. 1220–7, Jul. 2014.

[80] D. Bindreither, S. Ecker, B. Gschirr, A. Kofler, R. Kofler, and J. Rainer, 'The synthetic glucocorticoids prednisolone and dexamethasone regulate the same genes in acute lymphoblastic leukemia cells', *BMC Genomics*, vol. 15, p. 662, Jan. 2014.

[81] L. Seewald, J. W. Taub, K. W. Maloney, and E. R. B. McCabe, 'Acute leukemias in children with Down syndrome', *Mol. Genet. Metab.*, vol. 107, no. 1–2, pp. 25–30, Sep. 2012.

[82] A. S. Gamis, 'Acute myeloid leukemia and Down syndrome evolution of modern therapy--state of the art review', *Pediatr. Blood Cancer*, vol. 44, no. 1, pp. 13–20, Jan. 2005.

[83] M. C. Zwaan, D. Reinhardt, J. Hitzler, and P. Vyas, 'Acute leukemias in children with Down syndrome', *Pediatr. Clin. North Am.*, vol. 55, no. 1, pp. 53–70, Feb. 2008.

[84] Y. Ravindranath, 'Down syndrome and leukemia: new insights into the epidemiology, pathogenesis, and treatment', *Pediatr. Blood Cancer*, vol. 44, no. 1, pp. 1–7, Jan. 2005.

[85] Y. Ravindranath, 'Down syndrome and acute myeloid leukemia: the paradox of increased risk for leukemia and heightened sensitivity to chemotherapy', *J. Clin. Oncol.*, vol. 21, no. 18, pp. 3385–7, Sep. 2003.

[86] E. Hefti and J. G. Blanco, 'Anthracycline-related cardiotoxicity in patients with acute myeloid leukemia and Down syndrome: a literature review', *Cardiovasc. Toxicol.*, Jan. 2015. [Epub ahead of print].

[87] J. W. Taub, X. Huang, L. H. Matherly, M. L. Stout, S. A. Buck, G. V Massey, D. L. Becton, M. N. Chang, H. J. Weinstein, and Y. Ravindranath, 'Expression of chromosome 21-localized genes in acute myeloid leukemia: differences between Down syndrome and non-Down syndrome blast cells and relationship to in vitro sensitivity to cytosine arabinoside and daunorubicin', *Blood*, vol. 94, no. 4, pp. 1393–400, Aug. 1999.

[88] B. M. Frost, G. Gustafsson, R. Larsson, P. Nygren, and G. Lönnerholm, 'Cellular cytotoxic drug sensitivity in children with acute leukemia and Down's syndrome: an explanation to differences in clinical outcome?', *Leukemia*, vol. 14, no. 5, pp. 943–4, May 2000.

[89] C. M. Zwaan, G. J. L. Kaspers, R. Pieters, K. Hählen, G. E. Janka-Schaub, C. H. van Zantwijk, D. R. Huismans, E. de Vries, M. G. Rots, G. J. Peters, G. Jansen, U. Creutzig, and A. J. P. Veerman, 'Different drug sensitivity profiles of acute myeloid and lymphoblastic leukemia and normal peripheral blood mononuclear cells in children with and without Down syndrome', *Blood*, vol. 99, no. 1, pp. 245–51, Jan. 2002.

[90] Y. Ge, A. A. Dombkowski, K. M. LaFiura, D Tatman, R. S. Yedidi, M. L. Stout, S. A. Buck, G. Massey, D. L. Becton, H. J. Weinstein, Y. Ravindranath, L. H. Matherly, and J. W. Taub, 'Differential gene expression, GATA1 target genes, and the chemotherapy sensitivity of Down syndrome megakaryocytic leukemia', Blood, vol. 107, no. 4, pp. 1570–81, Feb. 2006.

Chapter 2

Leukemogenesis in Down syndrome

Ritsuko Shimizu and Masayuki Yamamoto

Additional information is available at the end of the chapter

http://dx.doi.org/10.5772/60598

Abstract

The incidence of leukemia is higher in Down syndrome children than that in the general population, while the risk of solid tumors is significantly reduced in Down syndrome. Recent studies utilizing mouse models have shown that distinct mechanisms caused by the elevated dosage of multiple genes is implicated in the protection from tumor progression depending on the type of solid neoplasm. In contrast, increased incidence of mutation in the several specific genes is reported as a cause of the onset of leukemias. Especially, acquired mutations in the *GATA1* gene are associated with leukemogenesis of megakaryoblastic leukemia (AMKL) and transient myeloproliferative disorder (TMD) related to Down syndrome. The mutations are clustered in the region corresponding to the N-terminal domain of GATA1 and result in the production of the short form of GATA1 (GATA1-S), which utilizes Met84 as an alternative translation initiation codon. Efforts producing mouse models of Down TMD and AMKL have been undertaken, as these models seem to provide important insights into the pathogenesis of multistep leukemogenesis. Concomitantly, the function of GATA1 has been examined extensively, and the analyses present a prototype for the study of lineage-restricted transcription factors that play an essential role for the differentiation, proliferation, and apoptosis of erythroid cells, megakaryocytes, mast cells, and eosinophils. In this chapter, we will summarize recent progress in the studies of leukemias that occur in Down syndrome, especially in relation to GATA1 mutations.

Keywords: Acute megakaryoblastic leukemia, Acute lymphoblastic leukemia, Transient myeloproliferative disorder, GATA1, Down syndrome

INTECH
open science | open minds

1. Introduction

The risk of solid tumors is significantly reduced in Down syndrome (DS) patients compared with the general population [1-3]. Studies utilizing mouse models have shown that distinct mechanisms caused by the elevated dosage of multiple genes are implicated in the protection from tumor progression depending on the type of solid neoplasm. In contrast, DS children have an increased risk of developing leukemias. Specifically, acute megakaryoblastic leukemia (AMKL) and acute lymphoblastic leukemia (ALL) are approximately 500 and 10-50 times more prevalent in children with DS compared to healthy controls, respectively [4-6].

Recent analyses have uncovered that a distinct pattern of acquired genetic mutations is implicated in the leukemogenesis restricted to DS children. In particular, acquired mutations in the *GATA1* gene are associated with leukemogenesis of DS-associated AMKL and transient myeloproliferative disorder (TMD), a preleukemic disorder unique to neonates with DS. The mutations are clustered in the region corresponding to the N-terminal domain of GATA1 and result in the production of a short form of GATA1 (GATA1-S), which utilizes Met84 as an alternative translation initiation codon. The function of GATA1 has been studied extensively, and the analyses present a prototype for the study of lineage-restricted transcription factors that play essential roles in the differentiation, proliferation, and apoptosis of erythroid cells, megakaryocytes, mast cells, and eosinophils. In this chapter, we summarize recent progress in the research on leukemias related to DS. Research of mouse models of DS TMD and AMKL has been undertaken, as these models seem to provide important insights into the pathogenesis of multistep leukemogenesis.

2. Unique features of leukemias associated with Down syndrome

There are substantial biological differences between the leukemias that occur in DS and non-DS children. It becomes increasingly clear that molecular mechanisms based on trisomy 21 affect not only the high incidence of leukemias but also the characteristic features of DS-associated leukemias.

2.1. DS-associated AMKL

Approximately 5-30% of DS babies are born with a leukocytosis with an erythroid-megakaryocytic immunophenotype. The severity of the clinical course varies with each case, from asymptomatic cases likely to have been considered peaceful births to severe cases resulting in critical injuries with blast cell infiltration of the organs. In severe cases, death from multiorgan failure or hepatic fibrosis is possible, requiring intensive care for the babies. Except for the most severe cases, symptoms usually resolve naturally (Figure 1). Therefore, DS-related leukocytosis is referred to as transient abnormal myelopoiesis (TAM) or transient myeloproliferative disorder (TMD). Patients suffering from TAM spontaneously achieve complete remission by 6 months of age. While the mechanisms of this spontaneous remission are still under investigation, one recent report showed that type I interferon signaling activated in bone marrow appears to attenuate the hyper-proliferation of megakaryocytes caused by the GATA1-S mutation [7].

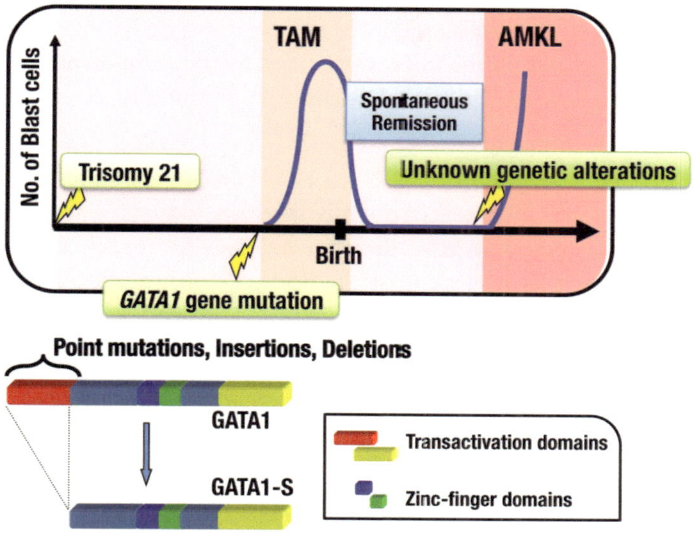

Figure 1. Multistep leukemogenesis of DS-associated AMKL. Megakaryocytic progenitors that have acquired various types of *GATA1* gene mutations eventually converge to GATA1-S, which develops TMD in DS fetus. The hyperproliferation phenotype of TAM blasts is canceled after birth. However, unknown genetic alterations transform the residual blasts to genuine leukemia.

After several years of asymptomatic periods, approximately 20% of DS children with a history of TAM develop genuine AMKL requiring intensive chemotherapy (Figure 1). It has been hypothesized that every DS child first diagnosed with AMKL has a history of asymptomatic TAM at birth. As a result, the incidence of AMKL in DS children is more than 500 times higher than in children without trisomy 21. Thus, this characteristic feature of DS-associated AMKL represents a potentially tractable model of multistep leukemogenesis. Chemotherapy in children with DS-associated AMKL shows a high cure rate. Therefore, the outcome of DS children with AMKL is statistically better than that of AMKL patents without trisomy 21 [8], probably due to the unique biological characteristics of blast cells. The molecular mechanisms of these remarkable differences remain as yet unknown.

In 2001, it was discovered that somatic mutations on the *GATA1* gene are frequently found in AMKL cases occurring in DS children [9]. Supporting evidence has appeared following the release of a paper describing the *GATA1* gene mutations found in TAM and DS-associated AMKL cases (Figure 1). Of note, the mutations are clustered in the region corresponding to the N-terminal domain of GATA1 and result in the production of the short form of GATA1 (GATA1-S) utilizing Met84 as an alternative translation initiation codon (Figure 1). A clinical study utilizing Guthrie blood shows that the *GATA1* gene mutation is found in the 3.8% of DS babies who are not diagnosed with TAM at their birth [10]. In some non-DS AMKL cases with the *GATA1* gene mutation, leukemic blasts originate from the cells that have somatically acquired trisomy 21 during myeloid development [11]. Similar cases are also observed in cells carrying trisomy 21 in mosaic models [12], suggesting that a cell-autonomous program provoked by the GATA1 mutation and trisomy 21 contributes to the onset of TAM. Relatively few cases of AMKL harboring mutations in the *GATA1* gene exist in the absence of trisomy 21 [13, 14]. Therefore, the pathogenesis of TAM seems to be closely associated with GATA1 dysfunction in combination with the impact provided by the extra chromosome 21. One of the important remaining questions is how DS children frequently acquire the *GATA1* gene mutation.

Sequential surveys of cases of TAM-AMKL have revealed that the type of *GATA1* gene mutations detected in AMKL blasts is frequently identical to that found in TAM blasts in each individual case, suggesting that AMKL develops in the TAM blasts. It seems plausible that TAM blasts survive during an asymptomatic period and some of the blasts receive additional hits and become genuine leukemic stem cell (Figure 1). Indeed, exome sequencings of TAM and AMKL blasts have revealed that the TAM blasts from one case have a singular *GATA1* gene mutation, while multiple mutations in the genes encoding for the cohesin components and epigenetic regulators are accumulated in the AMKL blasts in addition to the original mutation in the *GATA1* gene [15].

2.2. DS-associated ALL

Acute lymphoblastic leukemia (ALL) is one of the most common malignant diseases in children, and DS children have a higher incidence of this disease than non-DS children. In contrast to the DS-associated AMKL cases, the prognosis of DS-associated ALL is worse than ALL without DS. This may be because DS children are prone to suffer from significant toxicity of chemotherapy, as DS-associated ALL blasts retain high resistance against conventional chemotherapy regimens [16-18]. Intrachromosomal amplification of chromosome 21 (iAMP21) is also recurrently found in pediatric B cell leukemia, and this finding is considered to be an adverse prognostic factor [19, 20]. It has been demonstrated that target genes of the polycom repressor complex 2 (PRC2) are upregulated in both DS-associated ALL and ALL with iAMP21 [21], indicating that an epigenetic regulation provoked by trisomy 21 is a key mediator of the pathogenesis of this type of leukemia.

Mutations in the developmental genes for B-cell and T-cell lineages are often implicated in the pathogenesis of ALL, irrespective of the presence of Down syndrome. In addition to these genes, the incidence of mutations on genes involving the JAK/STAT pathway and RAS signaling have been found to be increased in DS-associated ALL [22-24], suggesting that molecular changes provided by these mutations may be the reason for the poor survival rate in children with DS-associated ALL.

3. Hematopoiesis in Down syndrome

It has been shown that hematopoietic homeostasis is significantly disturbed in DS fetus [25]. For example, frequencies of hematopoietic stem cells and megakaryocyte-erythroid progenitors are markedly increased showing high clonogenic characteristics, whereas that of granulocyte-macrophage progenitors is reduced [25-27]. In addition, committed pre-proB lymphoid and proB lymphoid progenitors are markedly reduced [25, 26]. This hematological abnormal-

http://dx.doi.org/10.5772/60598

ity may be a predominant cause of AMKL and ALL in DS babies. While the hematological abnormalities observed in newborns and infants with DS vary case by case, the following abnormalities are often observed: macrocytosis, neutrophilia, thrombocytopenia, and polycythemia [28-30]. In contrast to the high risk of leukemias in the pediatric period, leukemias are no longer a common cause of death in adults with DS [31]. Instead, macrocytosis and leucopenia are often observed in adult DS cases, leading to the early onset of myelodysplastic syndrome and bone marrow failure [32].

Strictly speaking, DS is defined by the possession of three copies of DS critical region (DSCR) of human chromosome 21 instead of two. However, the expression of genes located on chromosome 21 or the DSCR in DS patients is not always increased to 1.5-fold that of healthy controls. Depending on the expression levels, genes on human chromosome 21 or DSCR are divided into three categories: *i*) overexpressed genes, *ii*) genes expressed comparable to those in diploid healthy controls, and *iii*) genes whose levels are varied in individuals with DS. It has been reported that the frequency of genes overexpressed (type *i*) in B lymphocytes of DS patients is 22-39%, and the set of overexpressed genes in B lymphocytes differs from that found in fibroblasts [33, 34]. Therefore, it seems likely that the genes that proportionally increased due to the gene-dosage effect contribute to the common characteristic feature of DS, while the genes whose expression is varied in individuals determine the conditions of the individuals. In addition, microRNAs may be involved in the determination of DS disease types [35]. Expressional imbalances of chromosome 21-derived microRNAs may contribute to the diversified symptoms in DS patients.

To investigate the contribution of trisomy 21, three groups have independently established iPS (induced pluripotent stem) cells originated from DS patients and analyzed the hematopoietic differentiation. When iPS cells are cultured under the condition of primitive hematopoiesis (the first phase of hematopoiesis in yolk sacs), erythropoiesis is enhanced and myelopoiesis is reduced, while megakaryocytes are normally produced [36]. In contrast, when cultured under the condition of preferentially differentiating into fetal liver–derived definitive hematopoietic cells (the second phase of hematopoiesis in the fetal liver), iPS cells with trisomy 21 show increased multilineage colony-forming potential, and the number of cells with a myeloid and erythroid bipotential phenotype is increased [37]. However, trisomic iPS cells show no difference from isomic iPS cells when they are cultured in a condition suitable to generate erythroblast co-expressing embryonic and fetal globin genes [38]. Thus, the iPS studies suggest that the influence of one extra chromosome 21 to hematopoiesis is altered depending on the hematopoietic microenvironment.

Hematopoietic phenotypes have been examined in multiple lines of DS-model mice. Tc1 mice harbor an aneuploidy, carrying freely segregating human chromosome 21. The Tc1 mice show macrocytic anemia and an increased number of megakaryocytes with extramedullary hematopoiesis in the elderly. On the contrary, significant changes in frequencies of megakaryocytes, erythroid, and myeloid progenitors were not observed in the fetal liver [39]. Ts16 mice were generated by crossing mice with Robertsonian translocation Rb (14;16) and Rb (9;16), resulting in animals trisomic for mouse chromosome 16 (synthetic of human chromosome 21). Ts16 mice show increased erythropoiesis and reduced myelopoiesis during the embryonic period [40], but defects in hematopoiesis after the neonatal and infantile periods are uncertain, as Ts16 mice do not survive the postnatal period.

Ts65Dn, Tc1Cje, and Ts1Rh mice have been established as lines of euploid DS-model mice bearing a segmented region of mouse chromosome 16 containing 104, 81, and 33 genes, respectively. The Ts65Dn mice suffer from macrocytic anemia with defects of stem cell function and progressive myeloproliferative diseases [41]. In contrast, erythropoiesis is disturbed in Tc1Cje mice, but the mice never develop thrombocytosis or myeloproliferative diseases [42]. Hematopoietic analyses have been performed in Ts1Rhr mice, which are trisomic for the mouse equivalent of the hypothetical human DSCR; these mice show anemia and thrombocytosis in adulthood. Bone marrow cells of the mice preferentially differentiate toward the granulo-monocyte pathway, while the number of B cell progenitors is reduced [21, 43]. During the embryonic stage, hematological abnormalities are not found in Ts1Rhr mice, except for a significant increase in the hematopoietic stem cell population. Although each line of DS-model mice shows partially overlapping hematological phenotypes with those observed in patients with DS, none of the mice develop leukemia or acquire the *Gata1* gene mutation.

4. *GATA1* gene mutation in TAM and DS-associated AMKL

GATA1 is a founding member of the GATA family transcription factors that recognize consensus GATA binding motif. In mammals, the hematopoietic GATA subfamily is composed of GATA1, GATA2, and GATA3, which are expressed in erythroid and megakaryocytic cells, hematopoietic stem and progenitor cells, and T cells, respectively [44]. The expressions of GATA1 and GATA2 are partially overlapping, and these two GATA factors regulate the expression of each other. In early erythroid-megakaryocytic progenitors, GATA2 initiates *GATA1* gene expression, while GATA1 downregulates *GATA2* gene expression together with activation of its own gene expression [45]. We refer to this network regulation of GATA2 and GATA1 as GATA factor switching [45]. In addition, GATA1 and GATA2 share, at least in part, their target genes [46]. Consequently, GATA1 and GATA2 competitively or redundantly work for the expressions of their target genes dependent on the gene properties. Therefore, the functional balance of GATA1 and GATA2 is important for the maintenance of hematopoietic homeostasis.

The *GATA1* gene is composed of one untranslated first exon and five translated exons (Figure 2). The translation initiation codon located in the second exon is usually utilized to produce the full length of GATA1. Interestingly, an alternative splicing variant caused by the skipping of the second exon has been noticed in healthy humans, producing a short form of GATA1 protein lacking amino (N)-terminus 83 amino acids, which is identical to GATA1-S, utilizing an alternative translation initiation codon located in the third exon (Figure 2) [47]. In the case of mice, a short isoform of GATA1, a mouse ortholog of human GATA1-S, is also generated by the use of an alternative translation initiation codon in a single mRNA shared with the full-length of GATA1 [48]. Thus, two forms of GATA1 protein, GATA1 and GATA1-S, are both present simultaneously in healthy humans and mice, although the physiological roles of the GATA1-S isoform remain to be clarified.

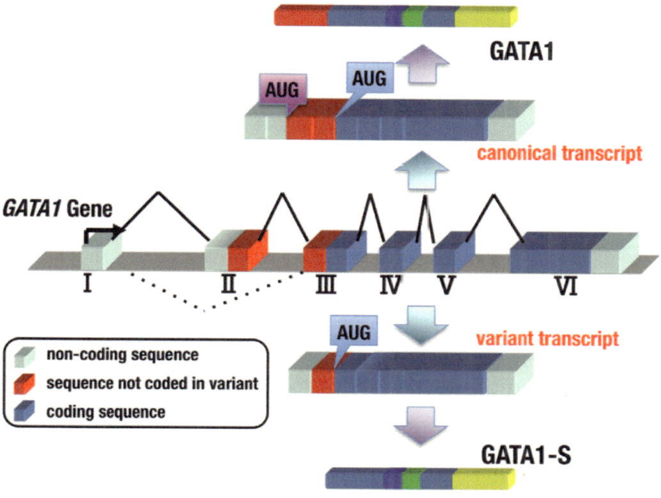

Figure 2. ***GATA1*** **gene construction and splicing variants.** *GATA1* gene is composed of an untranslated first exon and five translated exons. Full-length GATA1 is produced utilizing a translation initiation codon located in the second exon (upper panels). On the other hand, the GATA1-S variant is produced based on an alternative splicing variant, skipping the second exon and utilizing a methionine codon AUG corresponding to the 84th amino acid of full length of GATA1 (lower panels). Consequently, GATA1-S lacks the N-terminus 83 amino acids.

The *GATA1* mutations in TAM cases are clustered in the second exon of the *GATA1* gene, leading to the production of frame-shift misincorporation with the premature translation termination codon. Alternatively, mutations inducing pathological skipping of the second exon have also been reported [49]. Thus, the GATA1-S, but not the full-length GATA1, is exclusively produced in the TAM/AMKL blasts, indicating that aberrant function of GATA1-S in the absence of the expression of the full-length GATA1, rather than simple loss-of-GATA1-function, is involved in the onset of TAM.

GATA1 has four functional domains, two transactivation domains in the N- and carboxy (C)-terminal regions and two zinc-finger domains in the middle of body, which are important for the interaction with DNA and multiple cofactors (Figure 3A). Conventional cell-based luciferase reporter assays show that transactivation activity of GATA1-S is reduced into 30% of the full-length of GATA1, which is supported by the function of the C-terminal domain [50]. Functional analyses in mice *in vivo* indicate that the N-terminal and C-terminal transactivation domains differentially and cooperatively contribute to gene expression, depending on the property of GATA1 target genes. GATA1 target genes can be divided into three categories: the first group of genes requires only the N-terminal domain, the second group of genes requires only the C-terminal domain, and the third group of genes requires both domains [50]. The expression of only GATA1-S leads to the imbalance of GATA1 target gene expression, which may be implicated in the pathogenesis of TAM.

Importantly, provability of transformation into AMKL inversely correlates with the expression level of GATA1-S, and the latter is heavily dependent on the type of mutations in *GATA1* gene [48]. In the case of the mutations producing high amounts of GATA1-S, the incidence of AMKL is relatively low. However, such cases frequently suffer from high blast counts in the peripheral blood and require chemotherapy to prevent organ infiltration with the blasts. In contrast, patients with low amounts of GATA1-S frequently develop AMKL. Thus, the expression levels of GATA1-S influence leukemia progression and disease status.

Recently, two types of internally deleted (ID)-type GATA1 proteins were reported as a cause of TAM (Figure 3B) [51]. In the blasts of these cases, aberrant transcripts are produced due to splicing mutations in the *GATA1*, and, consequently, GATA1 proteins lacking amino acid residues 77-119 or 74-88 are produced. The N-terminal end of GATA1 is retained in the newly identified ID-type GATA1 mutants, while retinoblastoma protein (Rb)-binding motif LXCXE located around the Met84 is commonly deleted in GATA1-S and the ID-type GATA1 mutants (Figure 3B). Because binding potential with the Rb protein is important for the GATA1 functions of controlling cell proliferation and promoting erythroid differentiation [52], loss of the interaction with Rb protein may contribute, at least in part, to the GATA1 dysfunction leading to the pathological process of TAM.

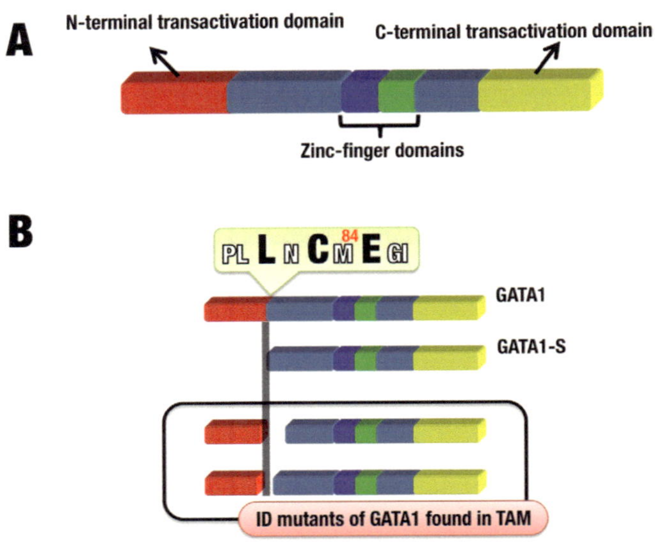

Figure 3. Rb-binding motif is commonly deleted in GATA1-S and the ID-type GATA1 mutants. A: domain structure of GATA1. Of note is that a pRb-binding motif LxCxE (aa 81-85) is commonly in wild-type GATA1. B: when the pRb-binding motif is eliminated in the GATA1-S and ID-type GATA1, the loss-of-function of the LxCxE motif appears to contribute to the TAM genesis.

5. Leukemogenesis caused by GATA1 deficiency

GATA1/Gata1 gene is located on the X chromosome in humans and mice. Hemizygous male mice with the *GATA1-null* germline mutation die *in utero* due to insufficient primitive erythropoiesis [53]. CFU-Meg (colony-forming unit-megakaryocyte) is significantly reduced in the yolk sac of *Gata1*-null embryos, indicating that GATA1 is indispensable for the primitive erythropoiesis and megakaryopoiesis. Independently, the *GATA1-knockdown* allele has also been constructed by inserting a neomycin resistance cassette just upstream from the first exon [54]. In this strain of mice, the strong promoter activity within the neomycin cassette directly interferes with the expression of the *Gata1* gene to approximately 5% of the wild-type level [54]. Hemizygous *Gata1-knockdown* mice also die *in utero*, showing a similar phenotype to the *Gata1-null* mice. These results indicate that 5% of the GATA1 level cannot support primitive erythropoiesis.

These two lines of *Gata1*-deficient mice have been maintained through heterozygous female mice. In female mice carrying the *Gata1* mutations, two types of hematopoietic progenitor cells are developed depending on the X chromosome inactivation. Hematopoietic progenitors with inactivated wild-type X chromosome and activated X chromosome with the *Gata1* mutation cannot differentiate into mature erythroid and megakaryocytic cells because of the defect in GATA1 function. In contrast, hematopoietic progenitors in which wild-type X chromosome is activated (and X chromosome with *Gata1* mutation is inactivated) differentiate normally to produce erythrocytes and platelets. Therefore, while *Gata1-null* and *Gata1-knockdown* heterozygous female embryos are anemic, these mice are born alive and grow normally.

However, interestingly, the female *Gata1-knockdown* mice frequently develop leukemia, while female *Gata1-null* mice never develop leukemia and have a normal life expectancy [55]. Characterization of leukemia cells shows that the cells are positive for c-Kit (a stem cell factor receptor) and CD71 (a transferrin receptor) antibodies but negative against the Ter119 (a molecule associated with glycophorin A) antibody. Further analyses have revealed that the leukemia is provoked by the residual 5% GATA1 in the immature erythroid progenitor cells carrying the activated *Gata1-knockdown* allele. In contrast, the progenitor cells with the activated *Gata1-null* allele never commit to leukemogenesis.

Because simple GATA1-deficiency causes a lethal embryonic phenotype, the roles of GATA1 in adult hematopoiesis are investigated using mice with conditional *Gata1* gene ablation. Adult *Gata1-null* mice produced by a conditional deletion of whole coding exons suffer from severe anemia and thrombocytopenia [56]. These mice lack erythroid progenitors, showing a phenotype resembling that of pure red cell aplasia. These results unequivocally indicate that GATA1 is required for erythroid commitment and erythropoiesis in the early stage of hematopoiesis. In addition, well-lobulated mature megakaryocytes that are positive for acetylcholine esterase (AchE) staining are accumulated in the hematopoietic organs of conditional *Gata1-null* mice, indicating that GATA1 is dispensable from the early stage of megakaryopoiesis and megakaryocyte development to matured polyploid megakaryocytes [56].

An additional line of GATA1-deficient mice (referred to as *Gata1*$^{\Delta IE}$) has been produced by a conditional deletion of the promoter/first exon of the *Gata1* gene [57]. The conditional adult *Gata1*$^{\Delta IE}$ mice also suffer from anemia. However, unlike the conditional *Gata1-null* mice, immature erythroid progenitors lacking terminal maturation potential to produce enucleated erythrocytes are accumulated in the hematopoietic organs of conditional *Gata1*$^{\Delta IE}$ mice. Also in these conditional *Gata1*$^{\Delta IE}$ mice, a small amount of aberrant *Gata1* transcript is produced in the erythroid progenitors utilizing alternative first exons located in the first and the second introns. These transcripts produce a small amount of GATA1-S, which supports the erythroid commitment of hematopoietic progenitors, but the cells fail to complete terminal erythroid maturation. In contrast, these aberrant transcripts are not produced in the megakaryocytes, and the megakaryocytic phenotype of the conditional *Gata1*$^{\Delta IE}$ mice is identical to that of the conditional *Gata1*-null mice.

We have generated germline *Gata1*$^{\Delta IE}$ mice by crossing the original flox mice with general Cre-expressing mice. It is worth noting that heterozygous female mice with the germline *Gata1*$^{\Delta IE}$ allele are prone to developing erythroleukemia, similar to the female *Gata1-knockdown* mice [58]. Thus, the impacts of changes in the expression level of GATA1 lead to the progression to leukemia in the mice, while the consequences also affect the erythroid differentiation differentially.

6. Mouse models of TMD and DS-associated AMKL

A transgenic complementation rescue approach has been successfully applied for the investigation of GATA1 function *in vivo*. Expression of full-length GATA1 under the transcriptional regulatory influences of *Gata1* recapitulates the GATA1 function *in vivo* and rescues various GATA1-deficient mice nicely from embryonic lethality [59]. Because transgene-derived mutant GATA1 is exclusively expressed in the rescued mice, one can reasonably expect that the phenotypes observed in the rescued mice occur due to the mutation.

Exploiting this rescue strategy, we have established transgenic lines of mice expressing GATA1-S. Transgenic expression of GATA1-S rescues the GATA1-deficient males from embryonic lethality [60]. Strikingly, immature megakaryocytes are accumulated in the fetal livers of the rescued mice, but this phenotype disappears after birth [61], indicating that the simple GATA1-S mutation provokes TMD-like phenotype in mice regardless of the presence of disomy or trisomy of chromosome 16 (the equivalent of human chromosome 21). In a colony-forming assay, progenitors with the GATA1-S mutation produced multiple progenies and generated enormously large colonies, consisting of innumerable immature megakaryocytes that were faintly positive for the AchE staining. In this assay, the number of CFU-Megs in the rescued embryos was equivalent to that in the wild-type embryos. Thus, GATA1-S failed to control proliferation and differentiation during the megakaryocyte differentiation process, resulting in an uncontrolled growth of immature megakaryocytes. It should be noted that TAM appears to be generated by single or a couple of hematopoietic progenitors acquiring the GATA1-S mutation, whereas in the rescued mice, all progenitors express GATA1-S. These observations suggest that the condition provided by trisomy 21 may lead to the onset of TAM by exploiting two pathways: one increases the frequency of GATA1-S mutation, while the other activates cellular mechanisms that magnify the impacts of the GATA1-S mutation.

One of the strong advantages of the transgenic complementation rescue assay is that levels of transgene-derived GATA1-S can be controlled. Because the expression levels of transgene-derived transcript vary between transgenic mouse lines depending on the integrated positions and/or copy numbers of the transgene, transgenic mouse lines expressing high-level GATA1-S and low-level GATA1-S have been used for the rescue analyses. The mice expressing high levels of GATA1-S never develop leukemia, whereas mice expressing low levels of GATA1-S are prone to developing leukemia. The leukemic cells have biphenotypic characteristics of erythroid and megakaryocyte lineages, closely resembling the human DS-associated AMKL (our unpublished observation). Thus, the expression levels of GATA1-S appear to be reflected in the transformation process of TAM blasts to genuine leukemia, consistent with the case of leukemogenesis in the erythroid progenitors of *Gata1-knockdown* mice caused by GATA1-deficiency.

Mice expressing GATA1 lacking N-terminal 63 amino acids have been established by gene targeting [62]. This line of mice showed transient hyper-proliferation of megakaryocytes in the fetal livers during the early stage of development, whereas the phenotype of the megakaryocytes in the later embryonic stages was close to normal. Because this mutant GATA1 molecule preserves the consensus Rb-binding motif, the effect of GATA1 mutation may be reduced. Another line of mice has been established by second exon deletion (*Gata1*$^{\Delta e2}$), and, consequently, only GATA-S is expressed in the *Gata1*$^{\Delta e2}$ mice [62]. This line of mice also shows transient hyper-proliferation of megakaryocytes during the early embryonic stage, similar to the GATA1 mutants lacking N-terminal 63 amino acids. In addition, the megakaryocyte progenitors derived from bone marrow of the adult *Gata1*$^{\Delta e2}$ mice are hyper-proliferative and formed significantly larger colonies than those in wild-type mice [7]. While the mechanism underlying the difference in the phenotypes of the rescued mice (hyper-proliferation of megakaryocytic progenitors until the perinatal stage [61]) and the *Gata1*$^{\Delta e2}$ mice (hyper-proliferation of megakaryocytic progenitors only in the early embryonic stages [62]) is unclear at present, these data congruently support the contention that the GATA1-S mutation alone gives rise to the hyper-proliferation of megakaryocytic progenitors in fetal mouse livers.

By crossing *Gata1*$^{\Delta e2}$ mice with DS-model lines of mice, *i.e.*, Tc1 and Ts1Rh, the contributions of GATA1-S mutation in combination with the trisomy of chromosome 21 to the leukemogenesis have been analyzed. The frequency of CFU-Megs in fetal livers is increased by the combination of *Gata1*$^{\Delta e2}$ and Tc1 mutations. However, this finding appears insufficient to provoke the onset of leukemia [39]. Similarly, when Ts1Rh mice are mated with *Gata1*$^{\Delta e2}$ mice, the compound mice did not show more phenotypes compared to the *Gata1*$^{\Delta e2}$ mutant mice in adulthood, except for further enlargement of megakaryocyte colony sizes [43]. The Ts1Rh and *Gata1*$^{\Delta e2}$ compound mutant mice never develop leukemia. However, intriguingly, bone marrow cells are prone to transformation into leukemic cells when MPL^{W515L} are retrovirally overexpressed in the compound mutant mouse cells [43]. MPL^{W515L} is an activating mutation of the thrombopoietin receptor, which is frequently found in patients with myeloproliferative neoplasms [63]. Therefore, it seems plausible that the megakaryocyte progenitors carrying the GATA1-S mutation become sensitive to the oncogenic mutation by the presence of trisomy 21. Thus, GATA1-S mutation in combination with trisomy 21 seems to give rise to the high transformation potential, which may be involved in the increased risk of leukemogenesis in DS children.

7. Conclusion

GATA1 is a lineage restricted transcription factor that is responsible for the hematopoiesis in erythroid and megakaryocyte lineages. GATA1 dysfunction leads to two types of leukemias. One type originates from the *quantitative deficit of GATA1,* which causes accumulation of immature erythroblasts and finally triggers erythroleukemia in mice [55]. The other type originates from the *qualitative defect of GATA1* (TMD and DS-associated AMKL) [64]. In the latter case, the GATA1-S mutation is provoked in high frequency, and the mutation contributes to the pathogenesis of TMD and DS-associated AMKL [49]. This structural change causes the accumulation of immature megakaryoblasts and finally triggers megakaryoblastic leukemia in mice and humans. Mice carrying a single GATA1-S mutation develop a phenotype resembling TAM [61]. In addition, trisomy 21 alters the function of hematopoietic cells [25-27], and in cooperation with GATA1-S, it leads to the pathogenesis of TMD and DS-associated AMKL. We surmise that the mouse models discussed in this chapter will provide important insights into the pathogenesis of TMD and DS-associated AMKL.

Acknowledgements

This study was supported in part by grants from JSPS (M.Y.), CREST program of JST and the Mitsubishi Foundation (to M.Y. and R.S.), and Friends of Leukemia Research Fund (R.S.). We also thank Ms. Aya Gotoh and Eriko Naganuma for their help.

Author details

Ritsuko Shimizu* and Masayuki Yamamoto

*Address all correspondence to: rshimizu@med.tohoku.ac.jp

Tohoku University Graduate School of Medicine, Sendai, Japan

References

[1] Hasle H, Clemmensen IH, Mikkelsen M. Risks of leukaemia and solid tumours in individuals with Down's syndrome. Lancet. 2000;355(9199):165-9.

[2] Sullivan SG, Hussain R, Glasson EJ, Bittles AH. The profile and incidence of cancer in Down syndrome. Journal of Intellectual Disability Research. JIDR. 2007;51(Pt 3): 228-31.

[3] Yang Q, Rasmussen SA, Friedman JM. Mortality associated with Down's syndrome in the USA from 1983 to 1997: a population-based study. Lancet. 2002;359(9311): 1019-25.

[4] Pui CH, Robison LL, Look AT. Acute lymphoblastic leukaemia. Lancet. 2008;371(9617):1030-43.

[5] Seewald L, Taub JW, Maloney KW, McCabe ER. Acute leukemias in children with Down syndrome. Molecular Genetics and Metabolism. 2012;107(1-2):25-30.

[6] Inaba H, Greaves M, Mullighan CG. Acute lymphoblastic leukaemia. Lancet. 2013;381(9881):1943-55.

[7] Woo AJ, Wieland K, Huang H, Akie TE, Piers T, Kim J, et al. Developmental differences in IFN signaling affect GATA1s-induced megakaryocyte hyperproliferation. The Journal of Clinical Investigation. 2013;123(8):3292-203.

[8] Lange BJ, Kobrinsky N, Barnard DR, Arthur DC, Buckley JD, Howells WB, et al. Distinctive demography, biology, and outcome of acute myeloid leukemia and myelodysplastic syndrome in children with Down syndrome: Children's Cancer Group Studies 2861 and 2891. Blood. 1998;91(2):608-15.

[9] Wechsler J, Greene M, McDevitt MA, Anastasi J, Karp JE, Le Beau MM, et al. Acquired mutations in GATA1 in the megakaryoblastic leukemia of Down syndrome. Nature Genetics. 2002;32(1):148-52.

[10] Pine SR, Guo Q, Yin C, Jayabose S, Druschel CM, Sandoval C. Incidence and clinical implications of GATA1 mutations in newborns with Down syndrome. Blood. 2007 ; 110(6):2128-31.

[11] Ono R, Hasegawa D, Hirabayashi S, Kamiya T, Yoshida K, Yonekawa S, et al. Acute megakaryoblastic leukemia with acquired trisomy 21 and GATA1 mutations in phenotypically normal children. European Journal of Pediatrics. 2014;10(1007):s00431-014,2430-3.

[12] Kudo K, Hama A, Kojima S, Ishii R, Morimoto A, Bessho F, et al. Mosaic Down syndrome-associated acute myeloid leukemia does not require high-dose cytarabine treatment for induction and consolidation therapy. International Journal of Hematology. 2010;91(4):630-5.

[13] Harigae H, Xu G, Sugawara T, Ishikawa I, Toki T, Ito E. The GATA1 mutation in an adult patient with acute megakaryoblastic leukemia not accompanying Down syndrome. Blood. 2004;103(8):3242-3.

[14] Hama A, Yagasaki H, Takahashi Y, Nishio N, Muramatsu H, Yoshida N, et al. Acute megakaryoblastic leukaemia (AMKL) in children: a comparison of AMKL with and without Down syndrome. British Journal of Haematology. 2008;140(5):552-61.

[15] Yoshida K, Toki T, Okuno Y, Kanezaki R, Shiraishi Y, Sato-Otsubo A, et al. The landscape of somatic mutations in Down syndrome-related myeloid disorders. Nature Genetics. 2013;45(11):1293-9.

[16] Buitenkamp TD, Izraeli S, Zimmermann M, Forestier E, Heerema NA, van den Heuvel-Eibrink MM, et al. Acute lymphoblastic leukemia in children with Down syndrome: a retrospective analysis from the Ponte di Legno study group. Blood. 2014;123(1):70-7.

[17] Zwaan CM, Kaspers GJ, Pieters R, Hahlen K, Janka-Schaub GE, van Zantwijk CH, et al. Different drug sensitivity profiles of acute myeloid and lymphoblastic leukemia and normal peripheral blood mononuclear cells in children with and without Down syndrome. Blood. 2002;99(1):245-51.

[18] Ragab AH, Abdel-Mageed A, Shuster JJ, Frankel LS, Pullen J, van Eys J, et al. Clinical characteristics and treatment outcome of children with acute lymphocytic leukemia and Down's syndrome. A Pediatric Oncology Group study. Cancer. 1991;67(4): 1057-63.

[19] Heerema NA, Raimondi SC, Anderson JR, Biegel J, Camitta BM, Cooley LD, et al. Specific extra chromosomes occur in a modal number dependent pattern in pediatric acute lymphoblastic leukemia. Genes, Chromosomes and Cancer. 2007;46(7):684-93.

[20] Moorman AV, Ensor HM, Richards SM, Chilton L, Schwab C, Kinsey SE, et al. Prognostic effect of chromosomal abnormalities in childhood B-cell precursor acute lymphoblastic leukaemia: results from the UK Medical Research Council ALL97/99 randomized trial. The Lancet Oncology. 2010;11(5):429-38.

[21] Lane AA, Chapuy B, Lin CY, Tivey T, Li H, Townsend EC, et al. Triplication of a 21q22 region contributes to B cell transformation through HMGN1 overexpression and loss of histone H3 Lys27 trimethylation. Nature Genetics. 2014;46(6):618-23.

[22] Bercovich D, Ganmore I, Scott LM, Wainreb G, Birger Y, Elimelech A, et al. Mutations of JAK2 in acute lymphoblastic leukaemias associated with Down's syndrome. Lancet. 2008;372(9648):1484-92.

[23] Mullighan CG, Collins-Underwood JR, Phillips LA, Loudin MG, Liu W, Zhang J, et al. Rearrangement of CRLF2 in B-progenitor- and Down syndrome-associated acute lymphoblastic leukemia. Nature Genetics. 2009;41(11):1243-6.

[24] Nikolaev SI, Garieri M, Santoni F, Falconnet E, Ribaux P, Guipponi M, et al. Frequent cases of RAS-mutated Down syndrome acute lymphoblastic leukaemia lack JAK2 mutations. Nature Communications. 2014;5:4654.

[25] Roy A, Cowan G, Mead AJ, Filippi S, Bohn G, Chaidos A, et al. Perturbation of fetal liver hematopoietic stem and progenitor cell development by trisomy 21. Proceedings of the National Academy of Sciences of the United States of America. 2012;109(43):17579-84.

[26] Tunstall-Pedoe O, Roy A, Karadimitris A, de la Fuente J, Fisk NM, Bennett P, et al. Abnormalities in the myeloid progenitor compartment in Down syndrome fetal liver precede acquisition of GATA1 mutations. Blood. 2008;112(12):4507-11.

[27] Chou ST, Opalinska JB, Yao Y, Fernandes MA, Kalota A, Brooks JS, et al. Trisomy 21 enhances human fetal erythro-megakaryocytic development. Blood. 2008;112(12): 4503-6.

[28] Henry E, Walker D, Wiedmeier SE, Christensen RD. Hematological abnormalities during the first week of life among neonates with Down syndrome: data from a multihospital healthcare system. American Journal of Medical Genetics Part A. 2007;143A(1):42-50.

[29] Hord JD, Gay JC, Whitlock JA. Thrombocytopenia in neonates with trisomy 21. Archives of Pediatrics & Adolescent Medicine. 1995;149(7):824-5.

[30] Miller M, Cosgriff JM. Hematological abnormalities in newborn infants with Down syndrome. American Journal of Medical Genetics. 1983;16(2):173-7.

[31] Englund A, Jonsson B, Zander CS, Gustafsson J, Anneren G. American Journal of Medical Genetics Part A. 2013;161A(4):642-9.

[32] McLean S, McHale C, Enright H. Hematological abnormalities in adult patients with Down's syndrome. Irish Journal of Medical Science. 2009;178(1):35-8.

[33] Ait Yahya-Graison E, Aubert J, Dauphinot L, Rivals I, Prieur M, Golfier G, et al. Classification of human chromosome 21 gene-expression variations in Down syndrome: impact on disease phenotypes. American Journal of Human Genetics. 2007;81(3): 475-91.

[34] Prandini P, Deutsch S, Lyle R, Gagnebin M, Delucinge Vivier C, Delorenzi M, et al. Natural gene-expression variation in Down syndrome modulates the outcome of gene-dosage imbalance. American Journal of Human Genetics. 2007;81(2):252-63.

[35] Shapshak P. Molecule of the month: miRNA and Down's syndrome. Bioinformation. 2013;9(15):752-4.

[36] Chou ST, Byrska-Bishop M, Tober JM, Yao Y, Vandorn D, Opalinska JB, et al. Trisomy 21-associated defects in human primitive hematopoiesis revealed through induced pluripotent stem cells. Proceedings of the National Academy of Sciences of the United States of America. 2012;109(43):17573-8.

[37] MacLean GA, Menne TF, Guo G, Scanchez DJ, Park IH, Daley GQ, Orkin SH. Altered hematopoiesis in trisomy 21 as revealed through in vitro differentiation of isogenic human pluripotent cells. Proceedings of the National Academy of Sciences of the United States of America. 2012;109(43):17567-72.

[38] Li LB, Chang KH, Wang PR, Hirata RK, Papayannopoulou T, Russell DW. Trisomy correction in Down syndrome induced pluripotent stem cells. Cell Stem Cell. 2012;11(5):615-9.

[39] Alford KA, Slender A, Vanes L, Li Z, Fisher EM, Nizetic D, et al. Perturbed hematopoiesis in the Tc1 mouse model of Down syndrome. Blood. 2010;115(14):2928-37.

[40] Gjertson C, Sturm KS, Berger CN. Hematopoietic deficiencies and core binding factor expression in murine Ts16, an animal model for Down syndrome. Clinical Immunology. 1999;91(1):50-60.

[41] Kirsammer G, Jilani S, Liu H, Davis E, Gurbuxani S, Le Beau MM, et al. Highly penetrant myeloproliferative disease in the Ts65Dn mouse model of Down syndrome. Blood. 2008;111(2):767-75.

[42] Carmichael CL, Majewski IJ, Alexander WS, Metcalf D, Hilton DJ, Hewitt CA, et al. Hematopoietic defects in the Ts1Cje mouse model of Down syndrome. Blood. 2009;113(9):1929-37.

[43] Malinge S, Bliss-Moreau M, Kirsammer G, Diebold L, Chlon T, Gurbuxani S, et al. Increased dosage of the chromosome 21 ortholog Dyrk1a promotes megakaryoblastic leukemia in a murine model of Down syndrome. The Journal of Clinical Investigation. 2012;122(3):948-62.

[44] Yamamoto M, Ko LJ, Leonard MW, Beug H, Orkin SH, Engel JD. Activity and tissue-specific expression of the transcription factor NF-E1 multigene family. Genes & Development. 1990;4(10):1650-62.

[45] Kaneko H, Shimizu R, Yamamoto M. GATA factor switching during erythroid differentiation. Current Opinion in Hematology. 2010;17(3):163-8.

[46] Suzuki M, Kobayashi-Osaki M, Tsutsumi S, Pan X, Ohmori S, Takai J, et al. GATA factor switching from GATA2 to GATA1 contributes to erythroid differentiation. Genes to Cells. 2013;18(11):921-33.

[47] Rainis L, Bercovich D, Strehl S, Teigler-Schlegel A, Stark B, Trka J, et al. Mutations in exon 2 of GATA1 are early events in megakaryocytic malignancies associated with trisomy 21. Blood. 2003;102(3):981-6.

[48] Calligaris R, Bottardi S, Cogoi S, Apezteguia I, Santoro C. Alternative translation initiation site usage results in two functionally distinct forms of the GATA-1 transcription factor. Proceedings of the National Academy of Sciences of the United States of America. 1995;92(25):11598-602.

[49] Kanezaki R, Toki T, Terui K, Xu G, Wang R, Shimada A, et al. Down syndrome and GATA1 mutations in transient abnormal myeloproliferative disorder: mutation classes correlate with progression to myeloid leukemia. Blood. 2010;116(22):4631-8.

[50] Kaneko H, Kobayashi E, Yamamoto M, Shimizu R. N- and C-terminal transactivation domains of GATA1 protein coordinate hematopoietic program. The Journal of Biological Chemistry. 2012;287(25):21439-49.

[51] Toki T, Kanezaki R, Kobayashi E, Kaneko H, Suzuki M, Wang R, et al. Naturally occurring oncogenic GATA1 mutants with internal deletions in transient abnormal myelopoiesis in Down syndrome. Blood. 2013;121(16):3181-4.

[52] Kadri Z, Shimizu R, Ohneda O, Maouche-Chretien L, Gisselbrecht S, Yamamoto M, et al. Direct binding of pRb/E2F-2 to GATA-1 regulates maturation and terminal cell division during erythropoiesis. PLoS Biology. 2009;7(6):e1000123.

[53] Fujiwara Y, Browne CP, Cunniff K, Goff SC, Orkin SH. Arrested development of embryonic red cell precursors in mouse embryos lacking transcription factor GATA-1. Proceedings of the National Academy of Sciences of the United States of America. 1996;93(22):12355-8.

[54] Takahashi S, Onodera K, Motohashi H, Suwabe N, Hayashi N, Yanai N, et al. Arrest in primitive erythroid cell development caused by promoter- specific disruption of the GATA-1 gene. The Journal of Biological Chemistry. 1997;272(19):12611-5.

[55] Shimizu R, Kuroha T, Ohneda O, Pan X, Ohneda K, Takahashi S, et al. Leukemogenesis caused by incapacitated GATA-1 function. Molecular and Cellular Biology. 2004;24(24):10814-25.

[56] Gutierrez L, Tsukamoto S, Suzuki M, Yamamoto-Mukai H, Yamamoto M, Philipsen S, et al. Ablation of GATA1 in adult mice results in aplastic crisis, revealing its essential role in steady-state and stress erythropoiesis. Blood. 2008;111(8):4375-85.

[57] Kobayashi E, Shimizu R, Kikuchi Y, Takahashi S, Yamamoto M. Loss of the GATA1 gene IE exon leads to variant transcript expression and the production of a GATA1 protein lacking the N-terminal domain. The Journal of Biological Chemistry. 2010;285(1):773-83.

[58] Shimizu R, Yamamoto M. Contribution of GATA1 dysfunction to multi-step leukemogenesis. Cancer Science. 2012;103(12):2039-44.

[59] Takahashi S, Shimizu R, Suwabe N, Kuroha T, Yoh K, Ohta J, et al. GATA factor transgenes under GATA-1 locus control rescue germline GATA-1 mutant deficiencies. Blood. 2000;96(3):910-6.

[60] Shimizu R, Takahashi S, Ohneda K, Engel JD, Yamamoto M. *In vivo* requirements for GATA-1 functional domains during primitive and definitive erythropoiesis. The EMBO Journal. 2001;20(18):5250-60.

[61] Shimizu R, Kobayashi E, Engel JD, Yamamoto M. Induction of hyperproliferative fetal megakaryopoiesis by an N-terminally truncated GATA1 mutant. Genes to Cells. 2009;14(9):1119-31.

[62] Li Z, Godinho FJ, Klusmann JH, Garriga-Canut M, Yu C, Orkin SH. Developmental stage-selective effect of somatically mutated leukemogenic transcription factor GATA1. Nature Genetetics. 2005;37(6):613-9.

[63] Pardanani AD, Levine RL, Lasho T, Pikman Y, Mesa RA, Wadleigh M, et al. MPL515 mutations in myeloproliferative and other myeloid disorders: a study of 1182 patients. Blood. 2006;108(10):3472-6.

[64] Shimizu R, Takahashi S, Ohneda K, Engel JD, Yamamoto M. GATA1-related leukaemias. Nature Review Cancer. 2008;8(4):279-87.

Chapter 3

Oral Health in Down Syndrome

Cristina Areias, Benedita Sampaio–Maia,
Viviana Macho, Ana Norton, Paula Macedo and
David Casimiro de Andrade

Additional information is available at the end of the chapter

http://dx.doi.org/10.5772/60652

Abstract

Oral health in Down Syndrome (DS) individuals has some peculiar aspects that must be considered in the follow up of these patients. In this chapter, we will focus on the oral and maxillofacial morphological alteration, the most prevalent oral pathologies as well as preventive measures and strategies for pathologies management in this population. Also, future research on oral health of DS will be discussed.

Keywords: Down syndrome, caries, periodontitis, saliva, microbiological and biochemical parameters, maxillary treatment, otorhinolaryngology, airway obstruction, pacifier-shaped device

1. Introduction

The skeletal and soft tissue features associated to DS individuals may contribute to increased drooling, angular cheilitis, dry mouth, and an increased prevalence and severity of fissured tongue and lower lips.[1-4] Bruxism (tooth-grinding) is a behavioural manifestation displayed by some DS individuals that may further contribute to alterations in tooth morphology and mineralization.[5-7]

Also, DS individuals have a significantly higher prevalence of some oral diseases, including periodontal disease, which develops at early age and is rapidly progressive as well as oral candidosis. [8-10] On the other hand, a lower prevalence of dental caries appears to be a characteristic of DS populations, although there are some controversial results.[11-15] The alteration in oral microbiology and biochemistry of DS population will be discussed in the light of these infectious diseases.[11]

However, the oral health problems experienced in people with DS are still not fully defined, so future studies are suggested.

2. Materials and methods

Bibliographic research undertaken through the MEDLINE/PubMed, Science Direct and B-on search engine as well as through the library archives of Porto University's School of Dental Medicine between 1988 and 2014 limited to articles published in English, French, Spanish and Portuguese. In total, 63 bibliographic references were obtained according to the following factors of inclusion: articles released by Porto University's School of Dental Medicine's servers through SCOPUS, ISI, Cochrane and PUBMED database, articles with titles referred in the keywords mentioned above.

3. Results and discussion

3.1. Maxillofacial and oral morphological features

Patients with DS have a high prevalence of specific otorhinolaryngologic pathology, including recurrent sinusitis and chronic nasal obstruction, as a consequence of hypotonia and craniofacial malformations (Figure 1.).[16-20]

The base of the skull, the frontal bone and the paranasal sinus are significantly small, leading to a decrease in the size of the sella turcica. There's a flattening of the cranial base as a result of vertical hypoplasia of the structures of the skull (Figure 1.).[2, 9, 17, 21]

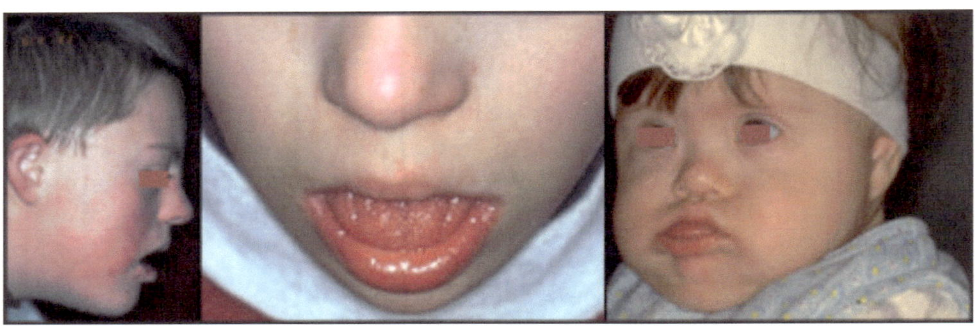

Figure 1. In DS, the respiratory dysfunction is among the pathologies that cause most worries and imply serious dysfunction in the individual development, learning ability and sleep capacity, as well as having large family repercussion.

http://dx.doi.org/10.5772/60652

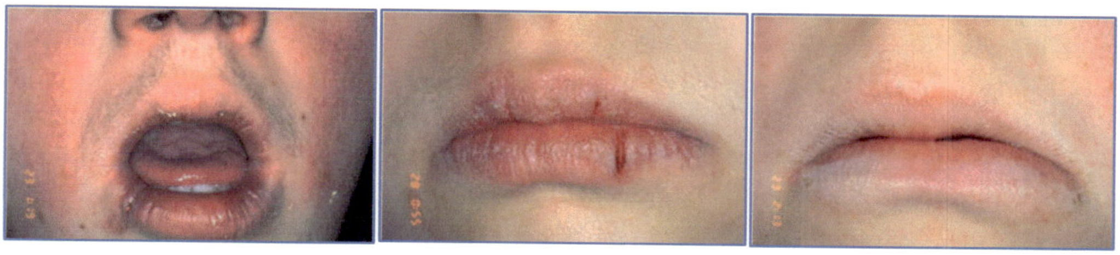

Figure 2. Dry skin and lips with fissures.

These problems, together with their short Eustachian tubes, predispose them to chronic media otitis with effusion and conductive hearing loss, which interferes with their language acquisition. They are also more susceptible to recurrent infections, particularly of the upper airway. [16-20]

Sleep apnea is diagnosed in more than 50% of the patients and may adversely affect behaviour, growth and neurodevelopment.[16, 20]

Another common abnormality is the dysfunction of the thyroid gland. Individuals with DS tend to present hypothyroidism and it is related to an underdevelopment of the bones and the teeth and to a delayed tooth eruption.[1, 2] The atlanto-axial joint, which is responsible for promoting communication between the first and the second vertebrae, is unstable in about 20% of the individuals.[1, 2] This defect may cause spinal cord compression during sudden movements of flexion and extension and, therefore, the dentist must be very careful while handling their necks.[1, 2]

When compared to the general population, these children have up to 20 times higher risk of developing leukaemia.[1, 2] The dentist should be alert to the presence of persistent lesions and spontaneous gingival bleeding as it may be an early sign of leukaemia.[3]

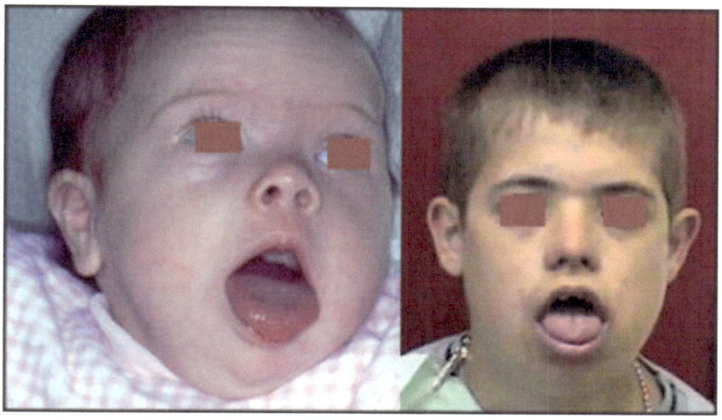

Figure 3. Some facial features of DS, to notice the hypotonia of facial muscles and tongue, with open mouth and tongue protrusion. Hypotonic lips, incomplete lip closure.

Mental health and behavioural problems, including attention deficit disorder, hyperactivity, obsessive-compulsive disorder and depression are common among individuals with DS.[9, 21, 22] Most of them also develop Alzheimer's disease around the fourth or fifth decade of life.[1, 2] This degenerative disease is related to an over-expression of β-amyloid precursor protein (βAPP), which is the expression of one of the triplicated genes in DS.[1, 2, 9] The most common craniofacial features observed in children with DS are small nose, low nasal bridge, narrow, short, deep and high palate, bifid uvula, hypertrophy of the tonsils, underdeveloped jaw, cleft lip, incomplete lip closure, hypotonic lips, fissured tongue, inaccurate and slow tongue movement, anterior open bite, posterior crossbite and reductions in the maxillary arch and changes in temporary and permanent tooth eruption (Figure 2., Figure 3., Figure 4., Figure5.).[6, 7, 9, 16, 17, 20, 23, 24]

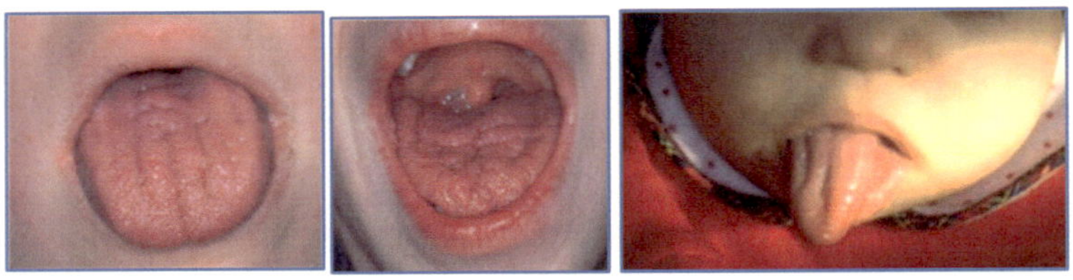

Figure 4. The scrotal tongue, sometimes with tongue diastasis, is often found in this syndrome.

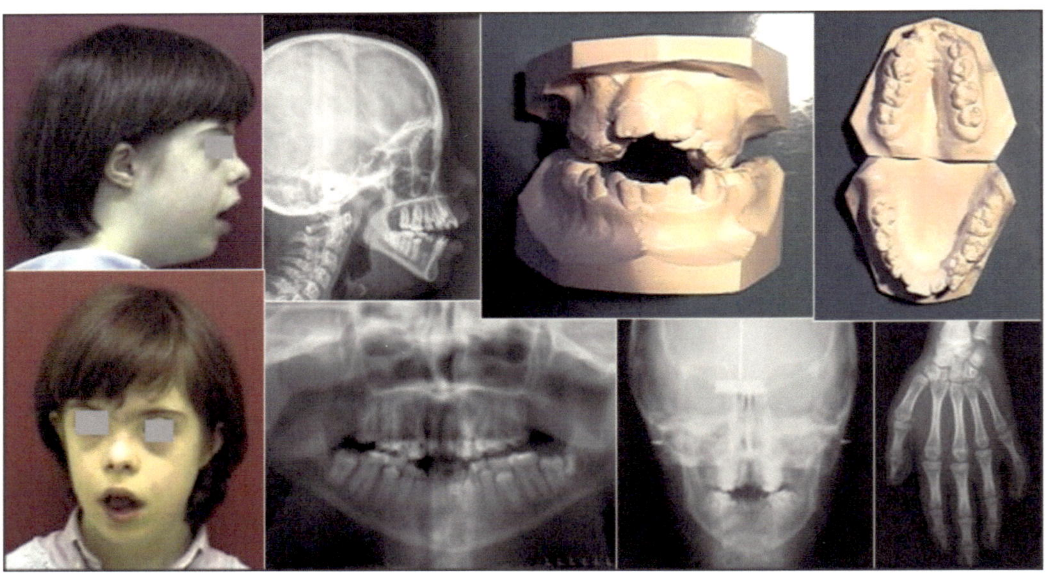

Figure 5. Lateral or anterior open bite is often found and tongue interposition worsens and maintains open bite.

This hypotonicity is associated with ligament laxity, easily visible throughout the body. It induces hyper-flexible joints, which can compromise the periodontal ligaments.[20] Excess of saliva on the labial commissure is also related to the muscle hypotonicity and can lead to irritation, cracking (angular cheilitis), aphthous ulcers and infectious conditions like candidiasis.[3, 24]

According to [Oredugba (25)], 51% of class I dental malocclusion and 47% of class III among 43 individuals with DS and only 5% of class III in the control group (individuals without DS), concluding that class III has a higher incidence in DS individuals than in the general population.

[Musich (26)] and [Soares K (27)] have concluded that class III is more frequent in DS individuals. Anatomically, the facial mid-third is underdeveloped but the mandible follows normal development (pseudo-progeny). This midface dysplasia also contributes to the narrow maxilla (Figure 5., Figure 6.).[7, 11, 18, 20]

Mandible measurements are not significantly different from normal subjects. However, a transverse expansion may occur due to lingual pressure.[20, 28] This intermaxillary discrepancy prevents the optimal intercuspal position to occur, which is needed to stabilize the mandible and the hyoid bone during mastication and swallowing.[16, 20]

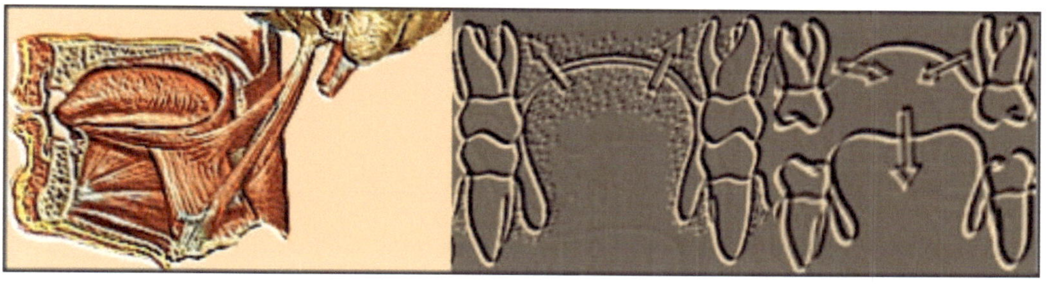

Figure 6. Natural position of the tongue, resting against the palate, creating a favourable force vector to maxillary growth; the protruded tongue and its low position, no longer exercises the vector of expansive force on the maxilla; on the other hand, the maintenance of the open mouth increases the compression.

Anterior crossbite is primarily attributed to the anteroposterior deficiency of the maxillary arch development, resulting in a crossbite of the mandible, projecting the jawbone arch towards the front of the maxilla (Figure 5., Figure 6.).[5, 6, 26-29]

Dental anomalies are very common, both in the primary and permanent teeth and occur with an incidence five times greater in DS individuals than in general population (Figure 7.).[7, 23]

Anomalies in the number (fewer), size (smaller) and morphology (crowns may also be short, small and conical) and the timing of their development (late dentition) are constant features of this syndrome.[7, 23] In the primary dentition, the most commonly absent teeth are lateral incisors, while in the permanent dentition, third molars, second premolars and lateral incisors, in this sequence, are the most frequently missing teeth (Figure 7.). [3, 7, 20]

Patients with DS have complete tooth mineralization, delayed tooth eruption (six to eighteen months) changes in the sequence of eruption (mainly of the temporary teeth), high incidence of impacted teeth (incisors and canines) and teeth agenesis. Microdontia, enamel hypoplasia, hypodontia of deciduous teeth and oligodontia are the most common dental anomalies. Structural abnormalities include taurodontia, peg-shaped teeth, fusion and germination. Canines are the most affected regarding shape and size.[3, 11, 20, 29, 30]

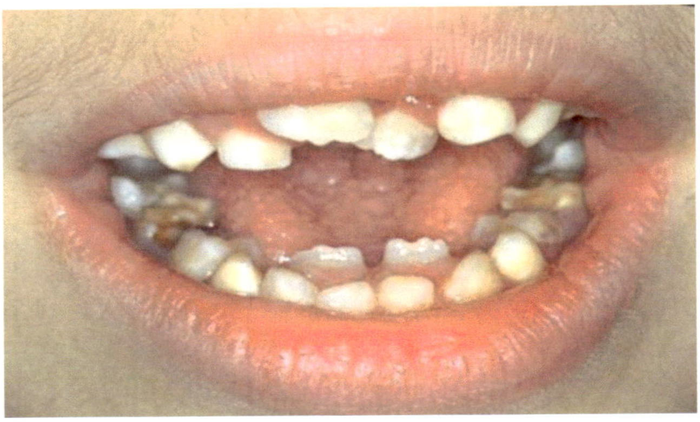

Figure 7. Delayed tooth eruption, compression and crowded teeth, microdontia, enamel hypoplasia, hypodontia of deciduous teeth and oligodontia.

3.2. Oral pathology

3.2.1. Caries

A majority of published studies have reported that people with DS have lower caries rates than people without DS, although several studies found that people with and without DS share the same caries rates, and some reported higher caries rates in those with DS.[7, 13, 14, 31] The differences herein described may be related to the control group used in each study: non-related healthy individuals, healthy siblings or other cognitive impaired individuals. The most commonly used indicator of caries experience is an index comprising disease and treatment markers, the DMFT (Decayed, Missing and Filled Teeth).[11, 12, 14] This index should be analysed together with factors such as a diet, frequency of snacking, social status, oral health in close relatives, dental awareness and past dental history. In studies of *Areias et al.* [11, 13, 14], the controls were sibling-matched, closest in age, in order to reduce the bias of factors like diet, social status and familiar oral health. In relation to DS, a more accurate assessment of caries experience risk is likely to be obtained by also examining the specific morphology. [32-34] The literature attributes the low prevalence of caries in individuals with DS to factors such as: eruptive pattern (teeth erupt later and so they are exposed to caries' etiological factors for less time); high prevalence of bruxism (flatter occlusal surfaces facilitate self-cleaning and oral hygiene, eliminating food debris that could be adhered to the sulcus and serve as a substrate for oral bacteria)[35]; dental morphology (microdontic teeth and diastema allow an early detection of caries with a simple clinical examination and without a radiological examination); salivary composition and differences in the composition of the microbiota (saliva buffer capacity of the individuals with DS appears to be higher when compared to general population); visit the dentist early in life (these children have several health problems and their parents seem to be easily warned of the oral risk factors).[11, 13, 14, 36, 37]

Saliva plays a crucial role in the defense against periopathogenic and cariogenic bacteria in the oral cavity and the equilibrium between demineralisation and remineralisation of enamel and dentin.[3, 12, 38] Consequently, the protective effects of salivary constituents, salivary flow rates and the salivary buffering capacity are essential.[36, 39-43] It is agreed almost universally that the salivary flow rate is significantly reduced in individuals with Down syndrome.[13, 36, 39-43] Also, *Siqueira et al.* [39] studied the whole unstimulated and stimulated saliva of people with Down syndrome for 2–5 years and found that salivary buffering capacity of these individuals is increased compared with healthy individuals of the same age. Regarding cariogenic microorganisms, it was reported that in adults and in children with trisomy 21, the lower caries rates was associated with lower levels of *Streptococcus mutans* in saliva.[13, 44] Besides the microbial factors, various salivary components are connected with the prevalence of caries.[45] The reduced saliva flow in DS individuals may be related to the existence of changes in the secretory function of the salivary glands of individuals with trisomy 21 and/or hypotonic muscle.[35, 36, 39-43, 45] Regarding the pH of the saliva of individuals with trisomy 21, there are some studies in which the values are higher [43] than ordinary people, while others have observed similar[11] or lower values.[39] There are several factors that could influence the results described in the literature, such as the analyses method (as used by each researcher), age of individuals, geographic location, food habits and time of collection. The buffer capacity of saliva is the ability to prevent changes in the pH of the environment (i.e. the buffer system is the major determinant of salivary pH). [36, 40, 43, 46] Salivary amylase is an important enzyme in the oral cavity. These authors showed low enzyme activity in individuals with trisomy.[40, 41, 46] *Areias C. et al.* [36] found in respect to α-amylases, the absolute salivary concentration as well as salivary secretion rate was similar between DS and sibling controls. IgA is the predominant immunoglobulin in saliva and which is produced by plasma cells of the salivary glands.[47] The IgA prevents microbial adherence, which can also justify reducing the prevalence of caries in children with Down syndrome.[45] A decrease in the levels of IgA in children with trisomy 21 (although not statistically significant) is explained by the onset of a state of immunodeficiency. [36] Other studies have shown differences concerning the IgA (higher in the group with Down syndrome).[40, 47] *Siqueira et al.* [40] showed that individuals with trisomy 21 have a greater concentration of protein in saliva, a fact that may be related to the low flow of saliva. Other ions analysed as zinc, magnesium, phosphorus and calcium showed no statistically significant differences between the group with Down syndrome and control group.[36]

3.2.2. Periodontal disease

The Gingivitis and Periodontitis are the two main subgroups of periodontal diseases affecting a high percentage of the world population and is therefore a serious public health problem.[8] Dental practitioners are challenged by the high incidence of early-onset aggressive periodontal disease in DS; these patients have higher levels of periodontal pathogens and periodontitis-associated interproximal bone loss. The complex anatomy, physiology, immunology and microbiology underscore the need for further investigation in specific areas related to dental treatment of these patients.[8, 48, 49] Gingivitis and periodontal disease start early in life, and the severity of these diseases increase with age. The prevalence of periodontal disease in adolescents with DS is 30% to 40%. Consequently, a large number of young people with DS lose their permanent anterior teeth in their early teens. In individuals in their thirties, the incidence of periodontal disease rises up to nearly 100%.[8] *Cichon et al. [8]*suggested that severe periodontal destruction that occurs in individuals with DS is compatible with aggressive periodontitis. Thus, periodontal disease is the most significant oral health problem in people with DS. The increased incidence of periodontal disease can be explained by the muscular hypotonicity and its consequences, dentoalveolar joint laxity, lack of understanding of the needs of oral hygiene, impaired dexterity, compromised immune system, low T cells count and leukocyte dysfunction. [31, 47, 48, 50, 51] Nutritional deficiencies can have an impact on periodontal health. Many studies have shown that there are a lot of nutrients that can have a negative impact on periodontal disease, but its wanted some vitamins, metals, antioxidants and proteins. [8, 49] By the time, only the deficiency in vitamin C and calcium and hyperlipidemia demonstrated significant results of increase risk in progression of the periodontal disease.[8, 49] Periodontal disease is induced by a complex microbiota, such as *Tannerella forsythia* and *Treponema denticola* (together called the red complex), which triggers intense inflammatory reaction. DS individuals demonstrate a high prevalence of periodontal disease compared with those who are otherwise chromosomally normal (euploids). [1, 49] Clinical parameters after non-surgical mechanical periodontal treatment were similar in diseased and healthy sites, independent of the genetic background.[10, 49] Diseased sites of DS and control patients harboured similar levels of *P. gingivalis* and *T. forsythia* at baseline, but significantly higher levels of *T. denticola* were found in DS patients. Increased levels of *P. gingivalis* at healthy sites were found in DS individuals. Non-surgical periodontal therapy decreased the levels of red complex microorganisms and improved the tested clinical parameters of diseased sites in both groups. However, the levels of red complex bacteria were higher in diseased sites of DS patients after the periodontal treatment.[10, 49] Although the mechanical periodontal treatment seemed to be effective in DS subjects over a short-term period, the red complex bacteria levels did not decrease significantly in diseased sites, as occurred in controls. Therefore, for DS patients, it seems that the conventional non-surgical periodontal therapy should be improved by utilising adjuvant to reduce the presence of periodontal pathogens.[10, 49]

3.2.3. Bruxism

Bruxism is quite common in this population, initiating at very young age, and often persisting throughout life. [5] The increased frequency of bruxism in DS population is associated to chronic anxiety, underdeveloped nervous system, malocclusion and TMJ dysfunction due to hypotonicity, hyper flexibility and laxity of the supporting ligaments. Initially, it creates an erosion of the pits and fissures of the occlusal surfaces (that become smoother), enabling self-cleaning with tongue and facilitating oral hygiene. [5, 11, 14] On the other hand, it can lead to an overloading of the supporting tissues and subsequent teeth fractures. These patients should be monitored through a regular program to allow an early diagnosis of the problems related to bruxism. [5, 14] In cases where bruxism is diagnosed, it is necessary to reposition the jaw and to decrease teeth grinding. Unfortunately, patients with a severe bruxism are the ones with more neurological problems and the treatment may not be successful.[5, 52]

3.3. Preventive and therapeutic intervention

This section intends to guide clinicians regarding the most important preventive measures in this population and also suggest the best approaches to improve the most common oral pathologies in DS individuals.[48] In this regard, oral hygiene and habits will be discussed and specific methods such as adapted DS pacifiers and rapid maxillary expansion will be suggested. According to *Areias C. et al.*, [11, 14] children with trisomy 21 start visiting the dentist before his brothers, probably due to increased parental concern. This may also explain the lower rate of DMF index found, considering that parents are first alerted to the need for effective oral health services.[11, 14] An appointment with the dentist regularly is important at all ages, but is essential in childhood and adolescence. In the study of *Macho V. et al.*, [6, 53, 54], the prevalence of occlusal anomalies found in mixed dentition was higher in the DS group than in their siblings. To improve the oral health of people with DS, health programs must incorporate intervention methods to control oral hygiene, to make Fluor and sealants application and to prevent and treat malocclusions as early as possible.[6, 53, 54] Therefore, there's a need to do a complete radiographic examination to identify hypodontia and other anomalies; occupational therapy to strengthen orofacial musculature; early mixed dentition orthodontic examination to screen for habits; and airway assessment, including consideration of tonsillectomy, palate expansion and tongue crib appliances (Figure 7., Figure 8., Figure 9. and Figure 10.). [16, 20, 24, 28, 55] Patients with DS should not be excluded from the general population with regard to dental care.[30, 56] From the ethical perspective, dentists must accept the responsibility and commitment to contribute with their knowledge to improve the quality of life of these people. Though children with DS can be excellent orthodontic patients, orthodontic prognosis may be poor because of their learning disability, parafunctional habits and severe periodontal disease (Figure 7., Figure 8., Figure 9. and Figure 10.). [16, 20, 24, 28, 55] The possible treatments of DS include prevention, interception or correction of the anomalies. We may find several actions during the different phases of growth: in early ages, and in the absence of teeth; in the temporary phase of teething; in the mixed phase of teething; in the definite phase of teething, up to the adult age. Orthodontic, orthopaedic and surgical approaches are possibilities of treatment. Complementary and peculiar approaches may include diminution of the size of the tongue, alteration from its position and increase of the space for the tongue – increase of the maxilla. To increase the maxilla, we may use techniques that produce first the bone growth or we modify the position of the muscles to orient the bone growth. These techniques are complementary and may be used in different ages. Each DS person is unique and it is fundamental that we always make an individualised study (Figure 8.).

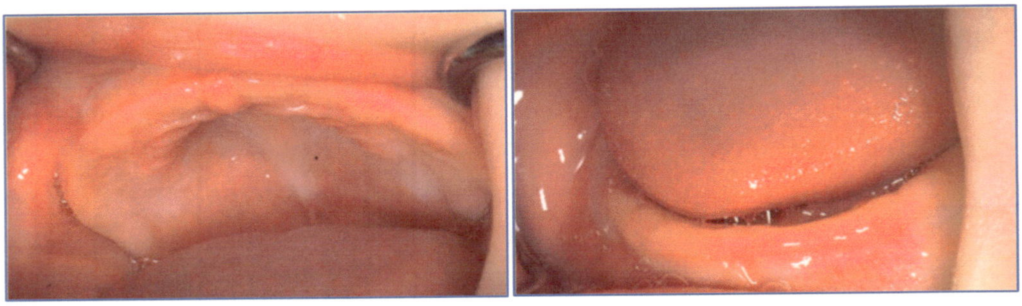

Figure 8. Baby mouth with Down syndrome.

3.4. Palatal plates

To improve the suction, drooling and the chewing and secondarily to help the development of the language, *Castillo-Morales* [57-61] developed a plate that consisted of an acrylic plate with many strategically placed accessories that stimulate different areas of the tongue, cheeks and lips, awakening reflexes that changed positions of different muscle groups (Figure 9.). The improvement of the health, face and the language favours the integration of the child with DS among the family and in society.[55] These plates have many benefits like give better respiratory characteristics, decrease in respiratory infections, improvement in sleep disturbance and improvement of bruxism. With the lingual re-establishment, it permits a better pronunciation of words and benefits aesthetically; secondly, it can even change the face of DS patients. The plate may be used for extended and repeated periods of the day, which contrasts with other stimulation methods (Figure10.).[57-61]In selected cases, a palatal plate is an excellent complement to traditional speech therapy and the most dominant factor for succeeding is motivation. [57-61]

After 12 months of therapy, the mean duration of the factor "closed mouth" was significantly longer ($p < 0.001$) and "inactive protrusion of the tongue" significantly shorter ($p < 0.001$) in the test group than in the control group. The results indicate that in children with Down syndrome, palatal plate therapy may be a valuable complement to a training program for improving orofacial muscle function. It may be used as a prophylactic measure of the tongue protrusion.

Undesirable effects after the insertion of the plate can occur; for example, development of active avoidance of the plate with the tongue, which results in more pronounced tongue protrusion, no clinical reaction, immediate habituation to the plate, hyper salivation or more pronounced tongue protrusion after the suspension of the treatment, even if for a short period.[57-62] All these reactions were rare, but required fitting a new plate, or suspension of the treatment.

Due to the presence of a protruding tongue and a muscular hypotonicity, these children have oral–motor problems (seen during swallowing, chewing and sucking) and are mouth breathers (exhibit open bite). The use of an adapted pacifier could prevent these problems (Figure 9).[3, 7, 11, 20]

http://dx.doi.org/10.5772/60652

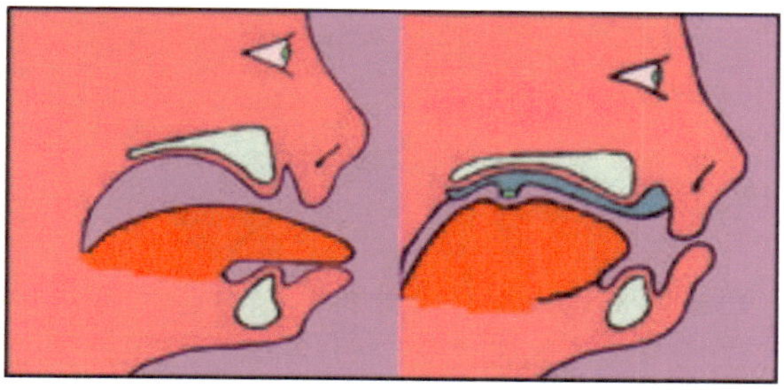

Figure 9. Reflex of Weiffenbach and repositioning of the tongue by the palatal plate.

When teeth are erupting, the plate does not adhere to the palate. So, they take off the plate easily, which leads to stopping the usage of the plate for a period until the child is about 3 years old. When the device is omitted for a period of time in the early stages of treatment, it will result in a return to the pathological condition. It is important to notice that people that already use the plates on their patients, don't refer major problems. Do not put plates if there is not a strong motivation by the parents. The motivation of the parents is fundamental.[57-62]

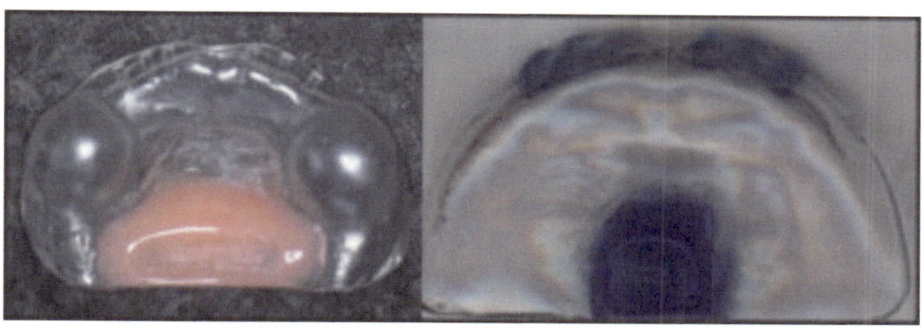

Figure 10. Examples of traditional palatine plates with tongue stimulat (a) or (in pink or in blue), and lip stimulatior(b)

Due to fear of plate swallowing and child choking, the plate developed by Castillo-Morales did not allow a prolonged use and required adult supervision [58]. Thereafter, Andrade C. et al [20, 63] developed a modified, pacifier-shaped device, that provide greater security, prolonged usage time (even at night), less concern by caregivers, and better acceptance by society. The results of its use show an improvement in aesthetics with less tongue protrusion and higher time of closed mouth when compared to the traditional Castillo-Morales plate (Figure 11., Figure 12., Figure 13.).[12, 20, 58, 63]

3.5. Fixed appliances

We can place fixed appliances in preschool age, if the child is cooperative. Problems like anterior or posterior crossbites should be corrected as soon as they are found. Fixed appliances have better results because we can have a greater control of their use, which does not happen with removable appliances, which can either be used or not. We may expand the maxilla to gain more space to the tongue and in DS we prefer to do it expanding from the apical base, to

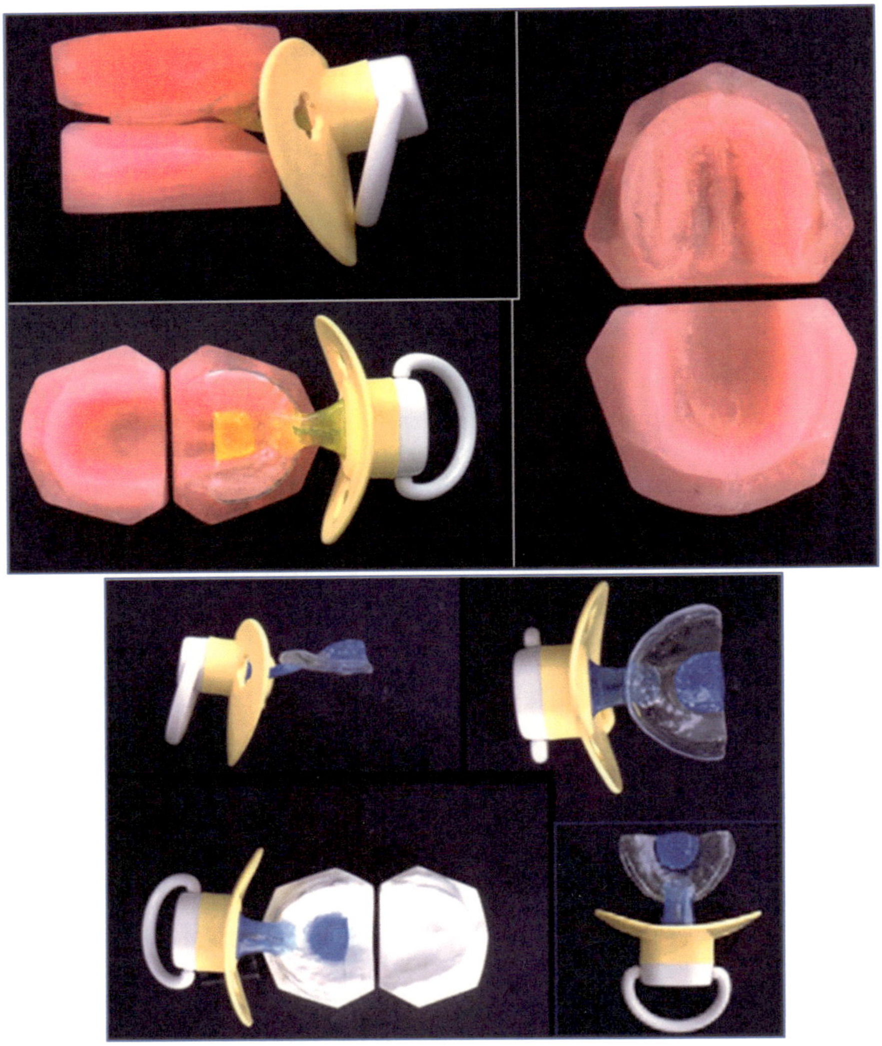

Figure 11. An alteration of the traditional plate now like a pacifier-shaped device.

obtain an orthopaedic effect. At certain ages, the effects of maxillary disjunction may be more favourable, which has to do with the overall growth of the jaws and the individual himself (Figure 13., Figure 14.). [20, 28]

Advantages of the device

- Fixed appliance
- Easy to clean
- Acts in a short time

http://dx.doi.org/10.5772/60652

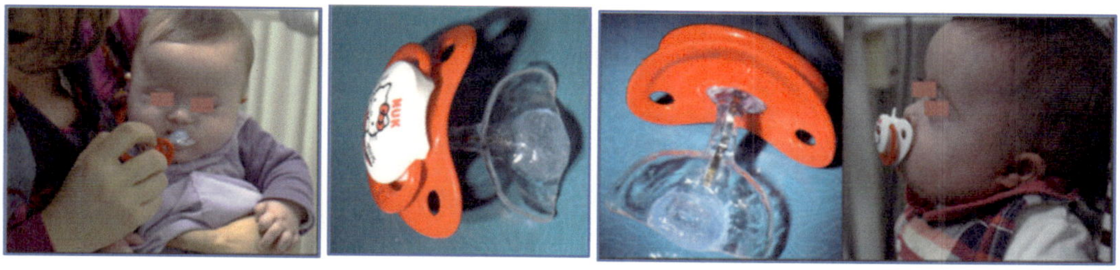

Figure 12. Pacifier-shaped device; the results of its use show an improvement in aesthetics with less tongue protrusion and higher time of closed mouth when compared to the traditional Castillo-Morales plate.

- Does not need intense cooperation from parents or from the children.

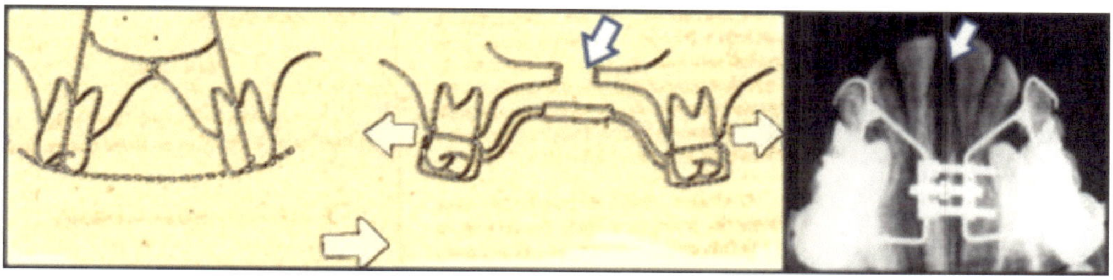

Figure 13. How to remove crossbites expanding from the apical base – the occlusal radiograph shows the disjunction of the maxilla; the superior incisors separated and the palatine suture opened.

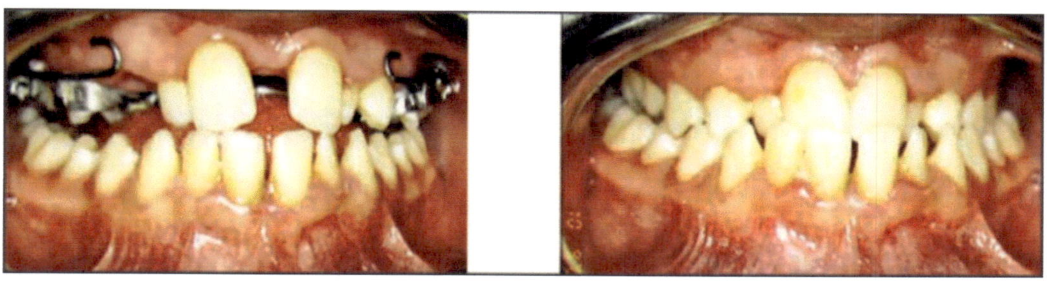

Figure 14. Effect of the maxillary disjunction in DS patient that presents bilateral and anterior crossbite. We open 0.3 to 0.5 mm a day, for 2 to 4 weeks.

Cutting this cycle of mouth breathing and increasing the area for nasal ventilation can provide a solution for some breathing difficulties, a reduction of tongue protrusion and drooling, as well as the high incidence of repeating respiratory infections and the high rates of compression and crossbites.[20, 28]

After the maxillary disjunction and in respect to clinical symptomatology, we may conclude:

Nasal symptomatology:

- Global improvement of cases and controls, but in that the cases show up, markedly, a minor incidence of rhinorrhea: "went the first summer in that my son had the nose completely without secretions".

Otologic symptomatology:

- Smaller evidence in the resolution from the serous otitis, that persisted in the cases and in the controls.

Rapid maxillary expansion produced a significant augmentation of nasal volume in children who had been treated ($p<0.05$) compared to the control group; these results were stable through the period of retention.

The rapid maxillary expansion (disjunction) in infants with Down syndrome:

- Diminishes the number of infections of the superior airways.
- Improves nasal permeability.
- Improves several parameters analysed by speech therapists.
- Tongue Mobility
- Articulation
- Intelligibility

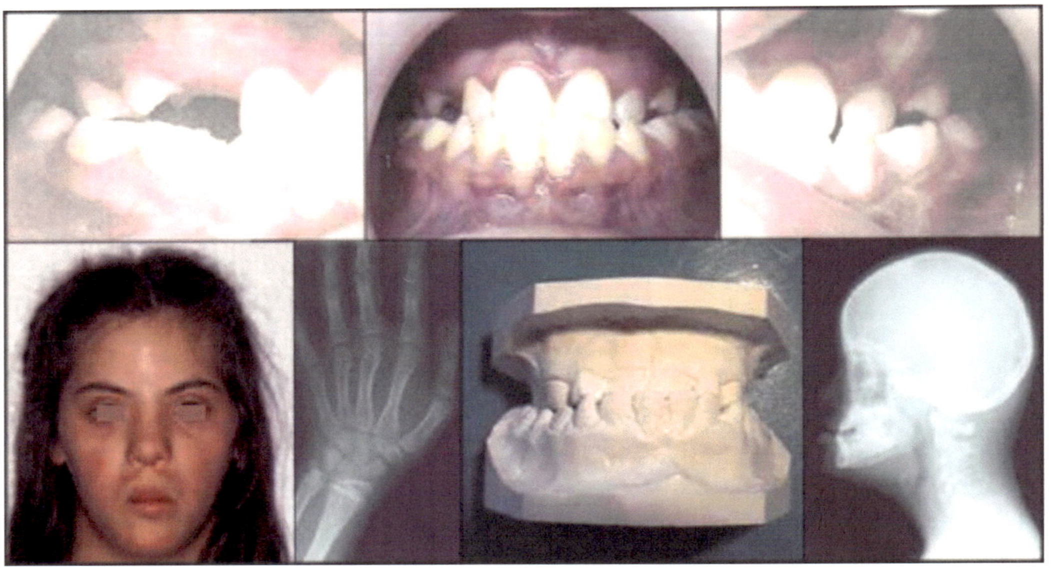

Figure 15. Patient with Down syndrome that present a bilateral crossbite (photographs extra and intra - orals, models and X rays).

http://dx.doi.org/10.5772/60652

Rapid maxillary expansion (RME) increased space for the tongue in the oral cavity (Figure 15., Figure 16., Figure 17.). This in turn results in a reduction of tongue protrusion and drooling. These aspects, in addition to the enlargement of the maxilla, often lead to an aesthetic improvement noted by the parents of the RME children. By placing the tongue in its normal position, the speech is improved, and so the aesthetics and self-confidence of the individual, facilitating his integration in society. This procedure may be carried out concomitantly with other surgical procedures for upper airway obstruction, sleep apnea and chronic otitis media with effusion. Rapid maxillary expansions give these patients a better airway, if used (Figure 15., Figure 16., Figure 17.). It is important to make exercise routines and teach these patients to use this new airway, increasing attention and activity, and leading to a better general development, better general health and less hours of work lost by the family. The indications should be accurate. The effect is similar to the infants from the general population. The use of this device should be included in the suggestion to medical and connected Associations of parents of Down's syndrome children.

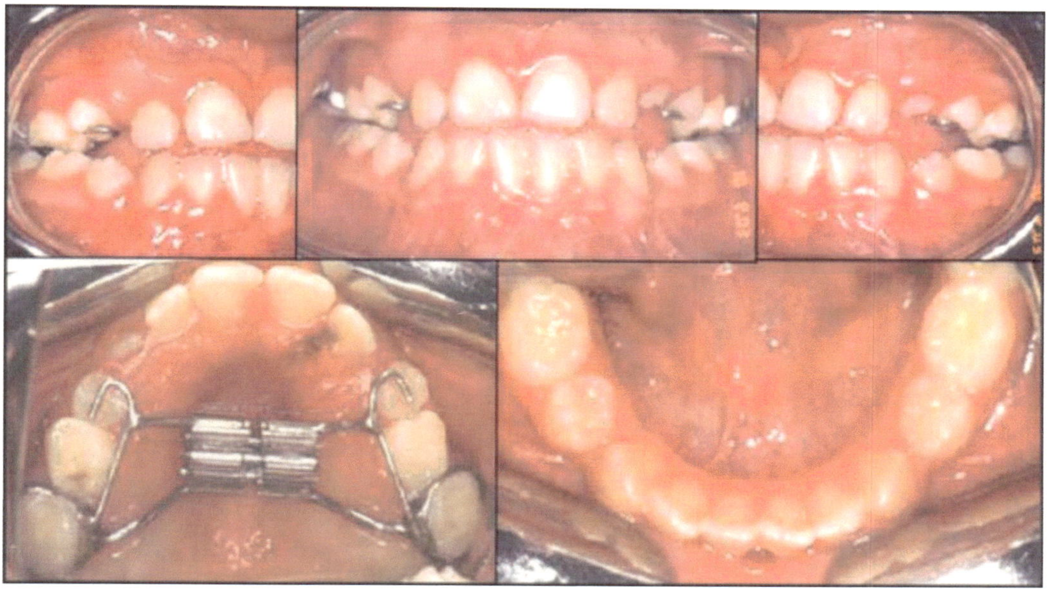

Figure 16. In less than one month, they obtain an increase from the apical base sufficient for eliminating the bilateral crossbite and the compression of the maxilla; this helps to facilitate the nasal ventilation.

We should not be afraid to use facial masks or other orthodontic devices because these patients are very supportive, and we should encourage all dentists to treat these patients.

We cannot forget that all cases must have an appropriate fixed orthodontic contention, in most times for life.The orthodontic retention phase minimises unwanted dental movements and maintains the corrections, and in these cases, most of the times, a fixed contention is necessary because hypotonia and deleterious habits are very dangerous for the stability of the correction (Figure 18., Figure 19., Figure 20., Figure 21.). [20, 28]

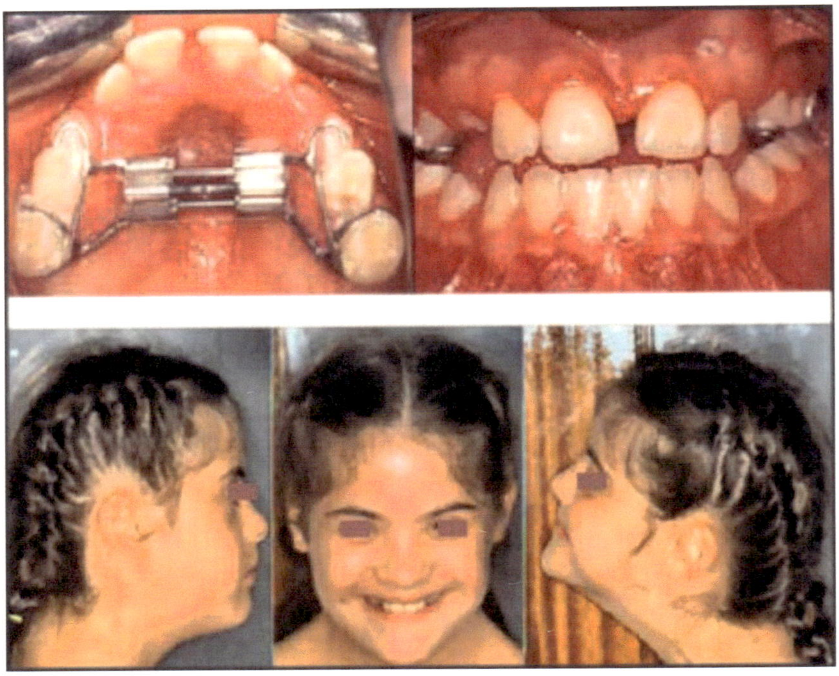

Figure 17. Immediately after rapid maxillary expansion; in addition to an aesthetic improvement observed by all parents, the beneficial effects of rapid maxillary expansion include better ventilation and drainage of secretions, which lowers the upper respiratory infections such as adenoiditis, tonsillitis and otitis verifying still an improvement of sleep apnea, decreased nasal obstruction and tongue protrusion.

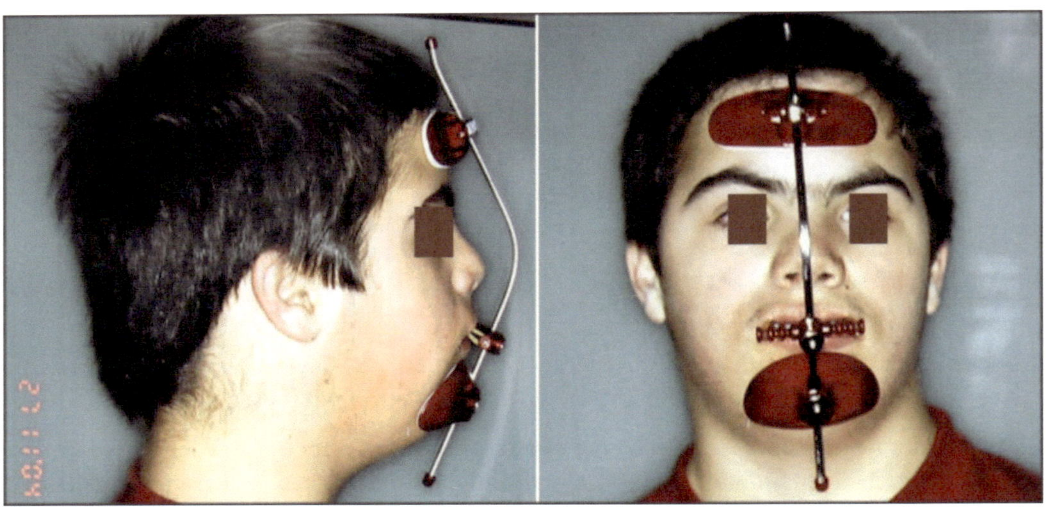

Figure 18. Facial mask may be used if necessary.

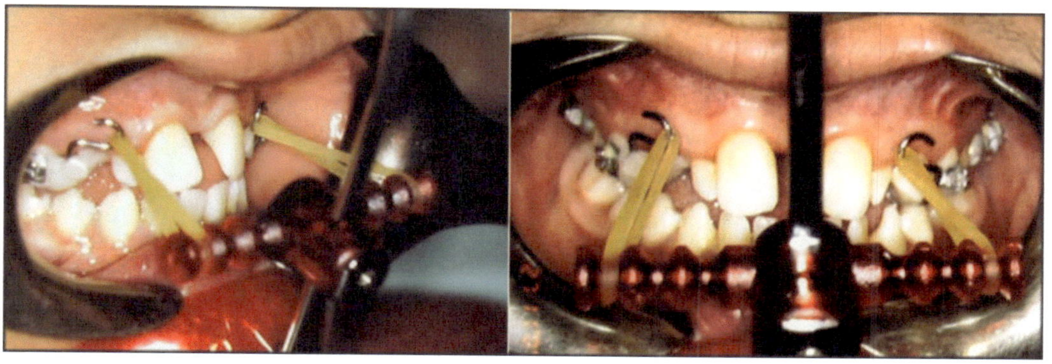

Figure 19. Facial mask immediately after disjunction.

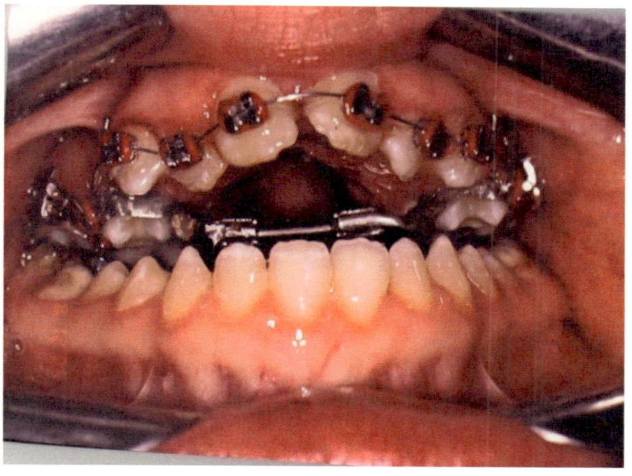

Figure 20. DS patients cooperate with the dentist and we should not be afraid to treat these patients.

4. Conclusion

Patients with Down syndrome present peculiar orofacial features that, when not corrected, may interfere with their physical, psychological and social development.

Children with this syndrome have a high risk of developing malocclusion and periodontal problems, and these should be the main concerns in their treatment needs. When planning the dental treatment of patients with Down syndrome, dental practitioners should always consider their general health, in order to achieve a holistic and interdisciplinary approach. Nevertheless, there is a need to improve the oral health services available to individuals with DS, to further investigate the interrelations between all their health problems, and to provide a higher level of information to parents of DS.

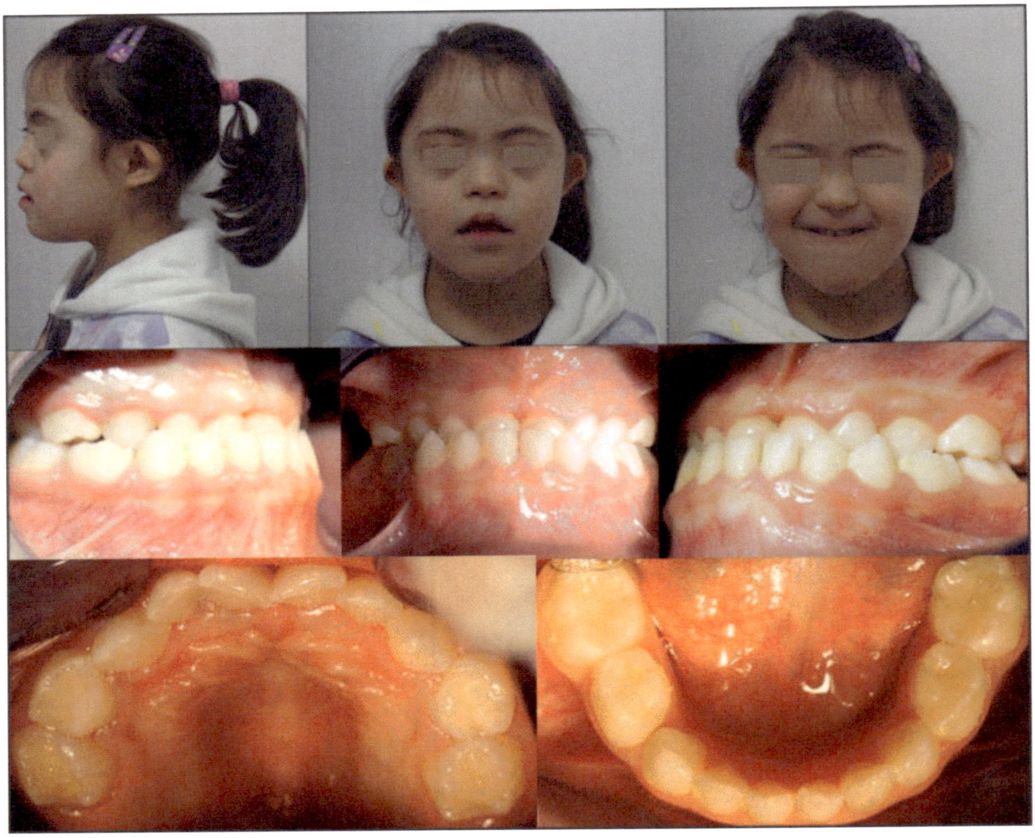

Figure 21. The crossbite may be present in primary dentition. If we have cooperation, we must correct the temporary teeth and not wait for the permanent teeth to get the treatment.

Acknowledgements

The authors supported this investigation.

Author details

Cristina Areias[1*], Benedita Sampaio–Maia[2], Viviana Macho[1], Ana Norton[1], Paula Macedo[1] and David Casimiro de Andrade[1]

*Address all correspondence to: careias@fmd.up.pt

1 Faculty of Dental Medicine of Porto University, Porto, Portugal

2 Faculty of Dental Medicine, INEB - Instituto de Engenharia Biomédica and Instituto de Investigação e Inovação em Saúde, Universidade do Porto, Portugal

The authors declare that they have no conflict of interest.
Cristina Areias, Benedita Sampaio-Maia: responsible for the conception and design.
Cristina Areias, Benedita Sampaio-Maia, Viviana Macho and Ana Norton were responsible for the data collection and manuscript redaction.
Benedita Sampaio-Maia and Paula Macedo were responsible for the critical revision of its contents.
David Casimiro de Andrade was responsible for graphics and photos and the critical revision of its intellectual contents and final approval of the version to be published.
All authors declare that written informed consent was obtained from the patient (or other approved parties) for publication of this research paper.

References

[1] Klug WS, Cummings MR, Spencer CA. Concepts of Genetics. Pearson Education, Upper Saddle River; 2006.

[2] Lewis R. Human Genetics Concepts and Applications, 7th ed. McGraw-Hill, New York; 2007.

[3] Shore S, Lightfoot T, Ansell P. Oral disease in children with Down syndrome: Causes and prevention. Community practitioner: The journal of the Community Practitioners' & Health Visitors' Association. 2010;83(2):18–21.

[4] Mouradian WE. The face of a child: Children's oral health and dental education. Journal of dental education. 2001;65(9):821–31.

[5] Macho V, Andrade D, Areias C, Norton A, Coelho A, Macedo P. Prevalência de hábitos orais deletérios e de anomalias oclusais numa população dos 3 aos 13 anos. Rev port estomatol med dent cir maxilofac. 2012;53(3):143–7.

[6] Macho V, Seabra M, Pinto A, Soares D, Andrade A. Alterações craniofacial e particularidades orais na Trissomia 21. Acta Pediatr Port. 2008;39(5):190–4.

[7] Macho V. Caracterização de uma população pediátrica com Trissomia 21: FMD-UP; 2007.

[8] Cichon P, Crawford L, Grimm WD. Early-onset periodontitis associated with Down's syndrome—Clinical interventional study. Annals of periodontology/the American Academy of Periodontology. 1998;3(1):370–80.

[9] Moreira Lília MA. A síndrome de Down e sua patogénese: Considerações sobre o determinismo genético. Rev Bras Psiquiatr. 2000;22(2):96–9.

[10] Martinez-Martinez RE, Loyola-Rodriguez JP, Bonilla-Garro SE, Patino-Marin N, Haubek D, Amano A, et al. Characterization of periodontal biofilm in Down syn-

drome patients: A comparative study. The journal of clinical pediatric dentistry. 2013;37(3):289–95.

[11] Areias C. Efeito da composição da saliva na prevalência cárie dentária em crianças com trissomia 21: Universidade do Porto Faculdade de Medicina Dentária; 2011.

[12] Vicente VA. Relação entre a prevalência da doença cárie e risco microbiológico. Cienc Odontol Bras. 2008;11(2):44–8.

[13] Areias C, Sampaio-Maia B, Pereira Mde L, Azevedo A, Melo P, Andrade C, et al. Reduced salivary flow and colonization by mutans streptococci in children with Down syndrome. Clinics. 2012;67(9):1007–11.

[14] Areias CM, Sampaio-Maia B, Guimaraes H, Melo P, Andrade D. Caries in Portuguese children with Down syndrome. Clinics. 2011;66(7):1183–6.

[15] Holst D, Schuller AA, Aleksejuniene J, Eriksen HM. Caries in populations—A theoretical, causal approach. European journal of oral sciences. 2001;109(3):143–8.

[16] Moura CP. Trissomia 21-Perspectiva Otorrinolaringológica. Arquivos de Medicina. 2004;18, 1/2: 61 - 65.

[17] Jacobs I, Gray RF, Todd N. Upper airway obstruction in children with Down syndrome. Arch Otolaryngol Head Neck Surg. 1996;122:945–50.

[18] Moura CP, Andrade D, Cunha LM, Tavares MJ, Cunha MJ, Barros H, Pueschel SM, Vaz P, Clemente MP. Down syndrome: Otolaryngological effects of rapid maxillary expansion. The journal of laryngology & otology. 2008;12(122):1318–24.

[19] de Moura CP, Andrade D, Cunha LM, Tavares MJ, Cunha MJ, Vaz P, et al. Down syndrome: Otolaryngological effects of rapid maxillary expansion. The journal of laryngology and otology. 2008;122(12):1318–24.

[20] Andrade DJ. Trissomia 21 – Estudo Dento-Maxilo-Facial FMD-UP; 2000.

[21] Fernandes A, Mourato P, Xavier M, Andrade C, Fernandes C, Palha M. Caracterização da evolução somática de crianças portuguesas com trissomia 21 – resultados preliminares. Acta Pediatr Port. 1998;29:261–8.

[22] Lewis CW, Grossman DC, Domoto PK, Deyo RA. The role of the pediatrician in the oral health of children: A national survey. Pediatrics. 2000;106(6):E84.

[23] Acerbi AG, de Freitas C, de Magalhaes MH. Prevalence of numeric anomalies in the permanent dentition of patients with Down syndrome. Special care in dentistry: Official publication of the American Association of Hospital Dentists, the Academy of Dentistry for the Handicapped, and the American Society for Geriatric Dentistry. 2001;21(2):75–8.

[24] Allison PJ, Hennequin M. The oral assessment in Down syndrome questionnaire (OADS): Development of an instrument to evaluate oral health problems in individuals with Down syndrome. Community dental health. 2000;17(3):172–9.

[25] Oredugba FA. Oral health condition and treatment needs of a group of Nigerian individuals with Down syndrome. Down's syndrome, research and practice: The journal of the Sarah Duffen Centre/University of Portsmouth. 2007;12(1):72–6.

[26] Musich DR. Orthodontic intervention and patients with Down syndrome. The angle orthodontist. 2006;76(4):734–5.

[27] Soares K, Mendes R, Junior R, Rosa L, Costa K. Prevalência de maloclusão em portadores de Síndrome de Down na cidade de Teresina-PI. Revista Gaúcha de Odontologia. 2009;57:187–91.

[28] de Moura CP, Vales F, Andrade D, Cunha LM, Barros H, Pueschel SM, et al. Rapid maxillary expansion and nasal patency in children with Down syndrome. Rhinology. 2005;43(2):138–42.

[29] Macho V, Coelho A, Areias C, Macedo P, Andrade D. Craniofacial features and specific oral characteristics of Down syndrome children. Oral health and dental management. 2014;13(2):408–11.

[30] Allison PJ, Hennequin M, Faulks D. Dental care access among individuals with Down syndrome in France. Special care in dentistry: Official publication of the American Association of Hospital Dentists, the Academy of Dentistry for the Handicapped, and the American Society for Geriatric Dentistry. 2000;20(1):28–34.

[31] Law V, Seow WK, Townsend G. Factors influencing oral colonization of mutans streptococci in young children. Australian dental journal. 2007;52(2):93–100; quiz 59.

[32] Fung K, Allison PJ. A comparison of caries rates in non-institutionalized individuals with and without Down syndrome. Special care in dentistry: Official publication of the American Association of Hospital Dentists, the Academy of Dentistry for the Handicapped, and the American Society for Geriatric Dentistry. 2005;25(6):302–10.

[33] Fung K, Lawrence H, Allison P. A paired analysis of correlates of dental restorative care in siblings with and without Down syndrome. Special care in dentistry: Official publication of the American Association of Hospital Dentists, the Academy of Dentistry for the Handicapped, and the American Society for Geriatric Dentistry. 2008;28(3):85–91.

[34] Gizani S, Papaioannou W, Haffajee AD, Kavvadia K, Quirynen M, Papagiannoulis L. Distribution of selected cariogenic bacteria in five different intra-oral habitats in young children. International journal of paediatric dentistry/the British Paedodontic Society [and] the International Association of Dentistry for Children. 2009;19(3):193–200.

[35] Tenuta LM, Ricomini Filho AP, Del Bel Cury AA, Cury JA. Effect of sucrose on the selection of mutans streptococci and lactobacilli in dental biofilm formedin situ. Caries research. 2006;40(6):546–9.

[36] Areias C, Sampaio-Maia B, Macho V, Leal I, Melo P, de Andrade C. Does the chemistry in the saliva of Down syndrome children explain their low caries prevalence? European journal of paediatric dentistry: Official journal of European Academy of Paediatric Dentistry. 2013;14(1):23–6.

[37] Catarina Barbosa JM, Milagre V, Andrade D, Areias C. Inhalation conscious sedation with nitrous oxide/oxygen in pediatric dentistry. MEDICALEXPRESS. 2014 Jun;1(3): 102-104

[38] Schaff-Blass E, Rozier RG, Chattopadhyay A, Quinonez R, Vann WF, Jr. Effectiveness of an educational intervention in oral health for pediatric residents. Ambulatory pediatrics: The official journal of the Ambulatory Pediatric Association. 2006;6(3):157–64.

[39] Siqueira WL, Bermejo PR, Mustacchi Z, Nicolau J. Buffer capacity, pH, and flow rate in saliva of children aged 2-60 months with Down syndrome. Clinical oral investigations. 2005;9(1):26–9.

[40] Siqueira WL, de Oliveira E, Mustacchi Z, Nicolau J. Electrolyte concentrations in saliva of children aged 6–10 years with Down syndrome. Oral surgery, oral medicine, oral pathology, oral radiology, and endodontics. 2004;98(1):76–9.

[41] Siqueira WL, Nicolau J. Stimulated whole saliva components in children with Down syndrome. Special care in dentistry: Official publication of the American Association of Hospital Dentists, the Academy of Dentistry for the Handicapped, and the American Society for Geriatric Dentistry. 2002;22(6):226–30.

[42] Siqueira WL, Siqueira MF, Mustacchi Z, de Oliveira E, Nicolau J. Salivary parameters in infants aged 12 to 60 months with Down syndrome. Special care in dentistry: Official publication of the American Association of Hospital Dentists, the Academy of Dentistry for the Handicapped, and the American Society for Geriatric Dentistry. 2007;27(5):202–5.

[43] Vijayaprasad KE, Ravichandra KS, Vasa AA, Suzan S. Relation of salivary calcium, phosphorus and alkaline phosphatase with the incidence of dental caries in children. Journal of the Indian Society of Pedodontics and Preventive Dentistry. 2010;28(3): 156–61.

[44] Lenander-Lumikari M, Loimaranta V. Saliva and dental caries. Advances in dental research. 2000;14:40–7.

[45] Davidovich E, Aframian DJ, Shapira J, Peretz B. A comparison of the sialochemistry, oral pH, and oral health status of Down syndrome children to healthy children. In-

ternational journal of paediatric dentistry/the British Paedodontic Society [and] the International Association of Dentistry for Children. 2010;20(4):235–41.

[46] Kavanagh DA, Svehla G. Variation of salivary calcium, phosphate and buffering capacity in adolescents. Archives of oral biology. 1998;43(12):1023–7.

[47] Lee SR, Kwon HK, Song KB, Choi YH. Dental caries and salivary immunoglobulin A in Down syndrome children. Journal of paediatrics and child health. 2004;40(9–10): 530–3.

[48] Cristina Areias VM, Coelho A, Pereira L, Andrade D, Pérez-Mongiovi D, Sampaio-Maia B. Enfoque clínico de niños con síndrome de Down en el consultorio dental. Avances en odontoestomatologia. 2014;(6):307-313.

[49] Tanaka MH, Rodrigues TO, Finoti LS, Teixeira SR, Mayer MP, Scarel-Caminaga RM, et al. The effect of conventional mechanical periodontal treatment on red complex microorganisms and clinical parameters in Down syndrome periodontitis patients: A pilot study. European journal of clinical microbiology & infectious diseases: Official publication of the European Society of Clinical Microbiology. 2015 Mar;34(3):601-8. doi: 10.1007/s10096-014-2268-7. Epub 2014 Nov 4.

[50] Cornejo LS, Brunotto M, Hilas E. Salivary factors associated to the prevalence and increase of dental caries in rural schoolchildren. Revista de saude publica. 2008;42(1): 19–25.

[51] Hennequin M, Allison PJ, Veyrune JL. Prevalence of oral health problems in a group of individuals with Down syndrome in France. Dev Med Child Neurol. 2000;42(10): 691–8.

[52] Martín M, Vasquez E, Diz P, Figueiral H, Vasconcelos L, Figueiredo J, Andrade D. Terapia de Estimulação Orofacial: Princípios e Considerações. Revista de Saúde Oral Revista de Saúde Oral. 1996;1:51–4.

[53] Macho V, Palha M, Macedo AP, Ribeiro O, Andrade C. Comparative study between dental caries prevalence of Down syndrome children and their siblings. Special care in dentistry: Official publication of the American Association of Hospital Dentists, the Academy of Dentistry for the Handicapped, and the American Society for Geriatric Dentistry. 2013;33(1):2–7.

[54] Macho V, Seabra M, Areias C, Ribeiro O, Andrade C. Comparação dos cuidados de saúde oral numa população com trissomia 21 e seus irmãos. Comparação dos cuidados de saúde oral numa população com trissomia 21 e seus irmãos. JADA. 2008;8(5): 2-14.

[55] Fischer-Brandies H, Limbrock GJ, Tragner-Born J. La Thérapie Fonctionnelle Sensorimotrice des Troubles Fonctionnels Oro-Faciaux Chez les Enfants avec I.M.C., d'après Castillo-Morales (Infirmité motrice cérébrale). L'orthodontie Française. 1988;59 Pt 2:449-58.

[56] Chung MH, Kaste LM, Koerber A, Fadavi S, Punwani I. Dental and medical students' knowledge and opinions of infant oral health. Journal of dental education. 2006;70(5):511–7.

[57] Carlstedt K, Dahllöf G, Nilsson B, Modeer T. Effect of palatal plate therapy in children with Down syndrome. A 1-year study. Acta Odontol Scand. 1996;54(2):122–5.

[58] Castillo-Morales R, Avalle C, Schmid R. Possibilità di Trattamento della Patologia Orofaciale nella Sindrome di Down con la Placa di Regolazione Motoria. Pediatria Preventiva e Sociale. 1984;34:1–4.

[59] Limbrock GJ, Castillo-Morales R, Hoyer H, Stover B, Onufer C. Castillo-Morales approach to orofacial pathology in Down syndrome. International journal of orofacial myology. 1993 Nov;19:30-7.

[60] Limbrock GJ, Fischer-Brandies H, Avalle C. Castillo-Morales' orofacial therapy: Treatment of 67 children with Down syndrome. Developmental medicine and child neurology. 1991;33:296–303.

[61] Limbrock GJ, Hoyer H, Scheying H. Regulation therapy by Castillo-Morales in children with Down syndrome: Primary and secondary orofacial pathology. Journal of dentistry for children. 1990 Nov-Dec;57(6):437-41.

[62] Hoyer H, Limbrock GJ. Orofacial regulation therapy in children with Down syndrome, using the methods and appliances of Castillo-Morales. Journal of dentistry for children. 1990;Nov–Dec:442.

[63] Andrade C, Tavares P, Rebelo P, Palha M, Tavares M. Placa modificada para tratamento de hipotonia oro-muscular em crianças com idade compreendida entre os 2 meses e os 2 anos. Ortodontia. 1998;3(2):111–7.

Section 2

Improvement of Cognitive Skills

Chapter 4

Assisted Cycling Therapy for Persons with Down Syndrome — Implications for Improvements in Cognitive Functioning

Shannon D. R. Ringenbach, Simon Holzapfel, Genna M. Mulvey and Sachin Pandya

Additional information is available at the end of the chapter

http://dx.doi.org/10.5772/60636

Abstract

To date, there are few, if any, behavioral or exercise interventions that have been shown effective in improving cognitive functioning in adolescents with Down syndrome (DS). Exercise is a logical answer because it has been repeatedly shown to improve cognitive and physical and mental health in typical populations. However, current exercise recommendations for persons with DS vary greatly. Recommendations are often nonspecific in terms of the type or intensity of exercise, and results on improvement of cognitive functioning are equivocal. This chapter will report on preliminary data of an 8 week intervention of assisted versus voluntary cycling exercise on cognitive and health functions in adolescents with DS. Assisted Cycling Therapy (ACT) is innovative and important because it is predicted to enhance neurogenesis, which in turn may improve multiple central nervous system functions related comorbid conditions in adolescents with DS.

Keywords: Executive function, aerobic exercise, activities of daily living, Alzheimer's disease, brain imaging

1. Introduction

Down syndrome (DS) is one of the most prevalent chromosomal conditions, affecting 1 in every 691 live births in the U.S.A. [1]. One of the main features of DS includes cognitive impairments.

Specifically, adolescents with DS have been shown to have lower levels on executive functions including working memory, inhibition, planning and set switching than typically developing children matched for mental age [2]. These cognitive deficits can limit their abilities to perform activities of daily living. Thus, interventions to improve their capacity to perform activities independently would help to improve quality of life and reduce the costs associated with providing care for them. We are investigating the effects of physical activity interventions on the cognitive skills in persons with DS.

1.1. Executive function

Executive functions are a set of higher-order control processes that take place primarily in the frontal lobe of the brain [2], which deal with the decisions to make actions, and planning how to accomplish tasks [3]. Executive function includes concept formation, task switching, inhibition, volition, planning, purposeful action, and effective performance [3]. These are necessary in order for a person to engage in tasks independently. People with deficits in executive function are often called lazy due to this lack of initiative, but executive function is necessary for a person to initiate self-care routines or work independently. Many researches have documented that people with DS have shown deficits in executive functioning (e.g., [4, 5]). Improving executive functions could in turn improve many other independent living skills. Below we have highlighted a few executive functions that we measured in response to an exercise intervention in persons with DS.

1.2. Working memory

Working memory is information that people actively keep in their mind and manipulate [3, 6]. If human memory were a computer, the working memory would have been an active window where a person would have manipulated the informational contents. Working memory is limited in size, yet it is important for many other tasks from remembering words to learning new motor skills [6, 7]. Several studies have found that people with DS have significant deficits in working memory [8, 9].

1.3. Set switching

Set switching is the ability to change a course of thought or action based on changing requirements [3]. In clinical settings, this is typically done with a card sorting test where children are first asked to sort the cards by shape and then by color. Children with typical development are unable to switch to the second sorting rule at three years old. By four years of age, a child can change rules with some struggle, and by five years old, a child can shift to the new rule with ease [10]. On a practical level, set switching is demonstrated while children are working on something when a parent tells them that they need to get ready to leave the house. The ease at which the children are able to transit between the two tasks reflects their capacity for set switching. Set switching also requires working memory to process the change in tasks and the ability to inhibit the first behavior pattern [11]. Set switching activates a network of cells in the frontoparietal region of the brain, including the inferior frontal gyrus, anterior cingulate cortex, and supramarginal gyrus [12]. When someone has difficulty with set switching, it can result

http://dx.doi.org/10.5772/60636

in inflexibility and perseverative behaviors. People with DS have significant deficits in set switching in comparison to people with typical development [2, 8].

1.4. Verbal fluency

People with DS in general show deficits with language, especially with expressive vocabulary [13–15]. Typically this is tested by asking people to recall words related to a particular category or words that start with a certain letter. Neuroimaging studies have shown that letter-based verbal fluency is mediated by the frontal cortex and category-based verbal fluency by the temporal cortex; parietal lobe mediates both tasks [16]. Nash and Snowling [17] found that people with DS showed deficits in verbal fluency in comparison with peers of typical development.

As previously described, there is a vast amount of research that documents cognitive deficits in persons with DS. We believe that it is time to focus on interventions aimed at improving cognitive functions in persons with DS. Our innovative exercise intervention and results will be explained next.

2. Intervention: Move fast, think fast

Exercise is a logical intervention for effective treatment of cognitive impairments in persons with DS because the positive influence of voluntary exercise on cognition has been demonstrated in other typical populations [18, 19], including children [20, 21] and older adults [22, 23]. Furthermore, voluntary exercise has been shown to improve memory in mice models (Ts65Dn) of DS [24]. However, a recent review of the therapeutic benefits of exercise in persons with DS found that exercise was nonsignificant in improving physical and mental health outcomes in persons with DS [25]. Because persons with DS move slowly [26] due to slower reaction times [27], deficits in muscular strength [28], and reduced cardiorespiratory capacity [29], adolescents with DS typically 'do' not exercise at a relatively high rate, 'thus, they miss out on the opportunity to gain' cognitive improvements through neuroplasticity in the brain. Furthermore, approximately 61% of persons with DS have been shown to have low exercise tolerance [30] which reduces their exercise time and intensity and which seems to limit the cognitive benefits of exercise for persons with DS [25]. The **voluntary aspect** of the exercise imposes major limitations in the quantity and quality of exercise in special populations such as those with DS.

There is an emerging body of literature in healthy older adults and individuals with Alzheimer's disease indicating that exercise results in structural and functional changes in the brain [31]. These alterations in brain structure and function suggest that CNS function can be altered via voluntary exercise in individuals with relatively normal and abnormal patterns of activation within the motor cortex. However, because persons with DS have limited motor output due to physiological and psychosocial factors, their ability to induce changes in CNS function may be compromised when engaging in voluntary exercise performed at their preferred (i.e., low) rates. They may need to have exercise augmented through mechanical assistance as proposed in our assisted exercise paradigm, coined Assissted Cycling Therapy (ACT) in 2013 [32]. Assisted exercise is an approach initially used with animals which were exercised on a motorized treadmill at a rate greater than their voluntary exercise rate. Assisted exercise has demonstrated improvements in cognitive functioning in animals [33] and most recently in patients with Parkinson's disease [34, 35]. ACT has been suggested to improve motor and cognitive function through its neuroprotective properties as demonstrated in Figure 1, a model proposed by Alberts and colleagues [34].

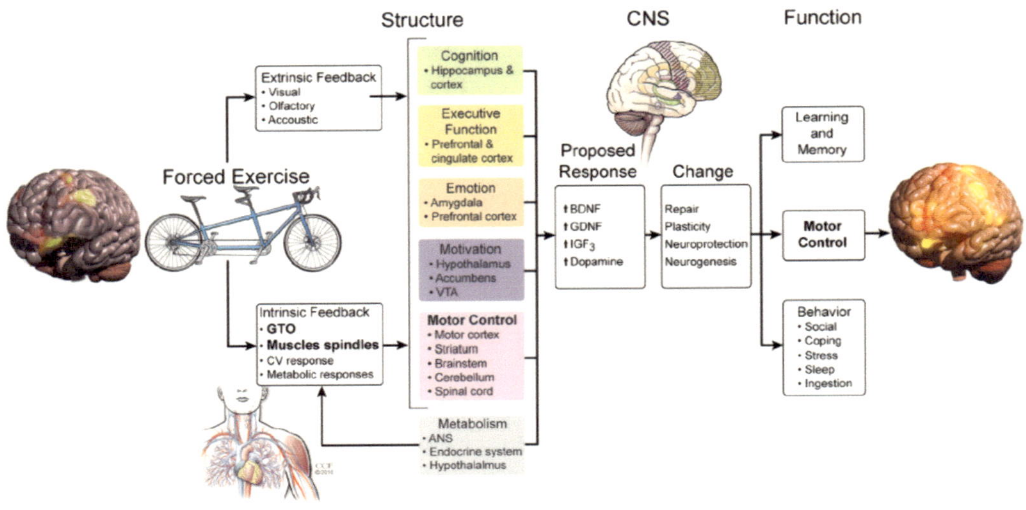

Figure 1. Proposed model for ACT (forced exercise) (Alberts et al., 2011).

2.1. Procedures for assisted cycling therapy

ACT is an emerging exercise paradigm especially suited for clinical populations who have limited voluntary movement output, exercise capacity, or exercise motivation. During ACT the electric motor of the bicycle is engaged which helps to increase pedaling cadence to a predetermined rate. We have used absolute cadences of approximately 80 rpm or relative cadences of 35% greater than the initial voluntary pedaling rate. The initial pedaling rates, however, may need to be increased gradually for comfort and familiarization. The ACT condition often leads to reduced power compared to voluntary pedaling as indicated in Table 1 by the lower average power contribution of our participants in the ACT condition than the voluntary cycling condition. As can be seen in Figure 2, special procedures were utilized to ensure that the feet were not positioned too far forward and that they did not slip forward, side-to-side, or backward to ensure a high degree of safety at the high pedaling rates.

The length of our intervention period was eight weeks with three cycling sessions per week. Before each cycling session, the resting heart rate (HR) was obtained while the participant was sitting on the bike. A five-minute warm up at a voluntary rate was completed before the 30-

http://dx.doi.org/10.5772/60636

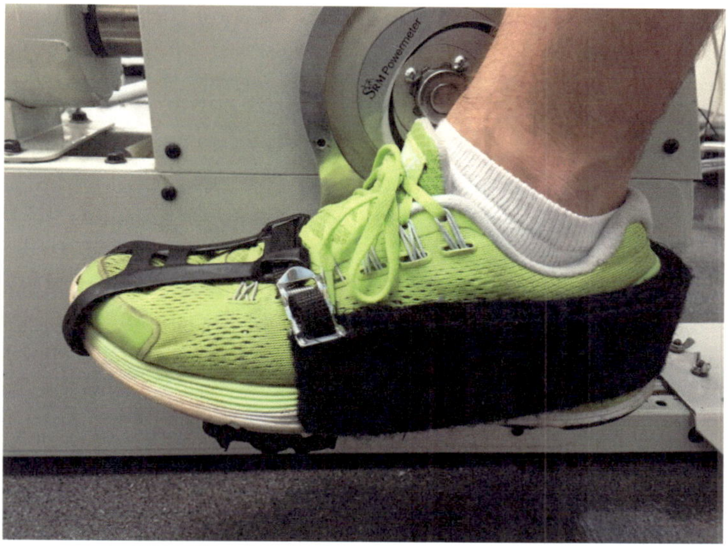

Figure 2. Pedal-foot interface.

minute cycling session regardless of the condition (ACT or voluntary cycling (VC)). On the first day, the average cadence from the warm-up period was multiplied by 1.35 to determine the initial ACT cadence. This step was omitted in the voluntary cycling condition. Thus, the cadence on the first day of the ACT intervention was set at a rate which was 35% faster than the voluntary cadence. A three- to five-minute cool-down at the end of the ACT or voluntary cycling session was optional. During the cool-down, the motor was not engaged. The average HR (bpm), cadence (rpm), and power (Watts) was recorded every five minutes during the cycling session (refer to Table 1 for mean values). These averages did not include the warm-up period.

To monitor Rate of Perceived Exertion (RPE), we used a modified -point RPE scale. A rating of 2 or 3 on the -point RPE scale (1, easy/not-tired; 2, a little hard/a little tired; 3, hard/tired; 4, very hard/very tired) was desired to keep the exercise intensity at a moderate level. The goal was for participants to cycle between 64 and 76% of their age-predicted maximal HR (HRmax = 210–0.56×age–31, [36]) which corresponds with a moderate exercise intensity as dictated by the American College of Sports Medicine [37]. Thus, for most participants in the ACT condition, we increased cadence from session to session by 3–5 rpm, based on tolerance, up to the maximum cadence of the motor (e.g., 95 rpm) or until 64% of age-predicted HRmax or a personal tolerance limit was reached. Participants in the ACT group took on average 13.2 cycling sessions to reach this point. Participants in the voluntary cycling group were not encouraged to pedal faster as the goal was to have them exercise at their preferred voluntary rate (refer to Table 1 for cadence values).

For this randomized control trial, participants were randomly allocated to eight weeks of ACT, eight weeks of VC, or eight weeks of no cycling (NC). The ACT and VC conditions were described in the previous section. Participants in the NC group completed only the pre- and posttesting sessions separated by eight weeks and they were instructed not to change their usual physical activity habits and therapy regiments for the eight weeks. Inclusion criteria consisted of trisomy-21 and a chronological age of 9–26 years. Exclusion criteria consisted of other genetic conditions and neurological disorders (e.g., ADHD and autism), medical contraindications to exercise, and sensory or physical impairments which preclude completion of the cycling intervention. During the pretesting sessions (first visit to the laboratory), the participants' height, weight, vision, hearing, and mental age were recorded or assessed. Mental age was determined with the Peabody Picture Vocabulary Test (4th ed.; [38]) (refer to Table 1 for chronological andmental age values). In addition, all participants had functional hearing and vision for the purpose of the testing procedures. Then, three executive function tests were administered in random order.

	ACT (n = 18)		VC (n = 16)		NC (n = 14)		One-way ANOVA
	Mean	**SD**	**Mean**	**SD**	**Mean**	**SD**	**p-value**
Chronological age (years)	19.4	4.9	18.4	3.4	17.0	4.0	0.304
Mental age (years)	6.1	3.3	5.2	2.1	6.0	1.8	0.687
BMI (kg/m^2)	27.7	7.0	27.3	4.2	27.5	9.5	0.889
Cadence (rpm)	77.2	2.2	43.1	8.9			<0.001'[1]
Power (Watts)	22.1	12.1	26.6	21.7			0.396'[1]
Heart rate (bpm)	98.7	8.0	100.7	7.7			0.642'[1]

[1] Independent samples t-tests were used to test group differences.

Table 1. Descriptive statistics

3. Measures

The verbal fluency test consisted of four categories: animals, food and drinks, words that start with an S, and words that start with an F. The participants were given one minute per category and had to name as many words in the category as possible. The verbal fluency test was a test of verbal long term and working memory, attention, and inhibition [39, 40]. As mentioned, verbal fluency and other speech and language deficits are well documented in persons with DS [41–43]. Verbal fluency tests have been used as behavioral measures of hippocampal and prefrontal cortex function [40, 43].

A backward digit span test was administered as a behavioral measure of working memory, which requires the simultaneous storage and processing of information [6, 44]. It is considered a prefrontal function [6]. During the backward digit span test, participants had to reverse a sequence of numbers given by the investigator. The investigator was providing progressively longer sequences of numbers until the participant could no longer accurately articulate the given sequence in reverse order.

http://dx.doi.org/10.5772/60636

The Wisconsin Card Sorting test (modified for DS) measures set switching ability and working memory which are functions of the frontal cortex and parts of the parietal lobe [45, 46]. In this task, the participants are asked to match either shapes or colors with rule changes taking place during testing. Adolescents with DS have been found to have reduced capacity for set switching compared to typically developing adolescents [2]. These three executive function tests were repeated during posttesting.

4. Results

Cohen's d effect sizes are considered small to medium if they range from 0.2 to 0.5, medium to large if they range from 0.5 to 0.8, and large if they are greater than 0.8 [47]. The effect sizes for the verbal fluency composite score were $d = 0.15$ for ACT, $d = 0.21$ for VC, and $d = 0.06$ for NC. The verbal fluency of the ACT and VC groups improved more than the verbal fluency of the NC group. The effect sizes for the backward digit span test were $d = 0.31$ for the ACT group, $d = 0.17$ for the VC group, and $d = 0.00$ for the NC group. The ACT and VC groups both showed improved working memory while the improvement was greatest in the ACT group. The effect sizes for the Wisconsin Card Sorting test were $d = -0.21$ for the ACT group, $d = 0.87$ for the VC group, and $d = 0.00$ for the NC group. Only the VC group improved in their set-switching ability. See Figure 3 for a visual representation of the results.

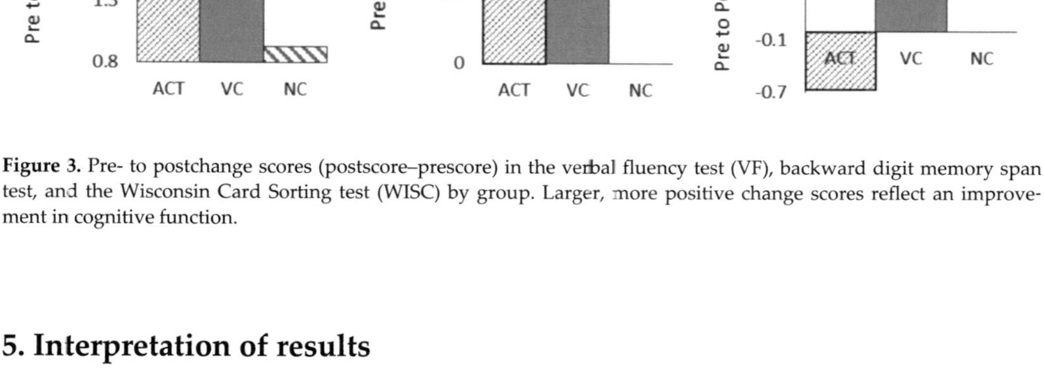

Figure 3. Pre- to postchange scores (postscore–prescore) in the verbal fluency test (VF), backward digit memory span test, and the Wisconsin Card Sorting test (WISC) by group. Larger, more positive change scores reflect an improvement in cognitive function.

5. Interpretation of results

It is clear that cycling exercise, whether it is assisted or voluntary, is more beneficial to executive function than no exercise. However, ACT seems to be more effective in improving working memory, whereas VC seems to be more effective in improving verbal long-term memory, and set switching than ACT.

Based on our results, a moderate exercise intensity, of between 64 and 76% HRmax, may not be necessary for benefits as the average HR during ACT or VC cycling sessions was just below 64% of the average age-predicted HRmax. The average chronological age of our participants in the ACT and VC group was 19.4 years and 18.4 years, respectively. This translates to minimum average target HRs (64%) of 107.6 bpm and 108.0 bpm in the ACT and VC group, respectively. In addition, their average exercising target HR of 98.7 bpm and 100.7 bpm were below the target HR range. In fact, on the first day of cycling, only 11% of ACT and 31% VC participants reached 64% of their age-predicted maximal HR. The only difference between the ACT and VC groups was the cadence at which they were cycling. We can thus conclude that the specific adaptations in terms of executive function are due to the different rates of movement.

The greater movement frequency during ACT would presumably lead to more frequent stimulation of the Golgi tendon organs and muscle spindle fibers in the lower extremity musculature and associated tendons, which in turn translates to greater afferent input to the frontal motor cortex [34]. This greater stimulus frequency in turn seems to be necessary to maximize benefits to working memory but does not seem necessary to improve long-term memory recall, attention, or set-switching ability. As can be seen in Table 1, heart rate s, and therefore cardiovascular workloads, were similar between ACT and VC, the only plausible explanation that remains for these group differences is the voluntary movement output during VC. The voluntary activation of certain areas of the motor cortex may thus be unique to voluntary exercise or greater in magnitude than the afferent stimulation resulting from ACT and thus benefit the frontal cortex in specific ways.

Differences in performance among executive function tasks, as observed in this study, have been documented [48]. Our results also suggest that different executive functions (e.g., working memory, attention, inhibition, and set-switching), though all mediated by the frontal cortex, may differentially benefit from different modes of exercise.

6. Future research

Our future research is to investigate whether exercise can prevent or slow the progression of Alzheimer's disease (AD) in persons with DS. AD is a serious dysfunction of global cognitive control, and adults with DS are at three to five times the risk of early onset of AD compared to the general population [5, 49]. AD is a neurocognitive degenerative disease that causes a loss of memory, thinking, and functioning abilities. It is known that as the lifespan of adults with DS increases, the prevalence of AD will rise concomitantly. However, there is not much research in this area [50]. Research in this field can be aimed toward the development of an intervention, as well as prevention of AD in patients with DS. In order to reach that status, there must be more involvement of the DS population into clinical trials so that sufficient data can be collected and analyzed.

In addition, brain imaging is an important tool and is used in both clinical diagnosis and in the research of AD in persons with DS. In this research, many different types of imaging techniques are used to determine participant eligibility as well as to test if the imaging can accurately predict the participant's risk of developing AD. These imaging techniques include, but are not limited to, amyloid PET scans, functional MRIs, structural MRIs, and CTs [51]. Each type of imaging will provide a view into the different mechanisms leading to the development of AD. Amyloid PET scans are a type of positron emission tomography in which amyloid plaque is targeted with radioactive tracers to be seen on the image. It is thought that an abnormal amount of these plaques predisposes the participant to developing AD. While this type of imaging is futile in the clinical setting, researchers can choose to look for participants who have this abnormal amount of amyloid plaque but show no symptoms, so that an intervention can be created for those individuals. MRIs and CTs have more impact in the clinical setting because they focus on the structure of the brain. Research has shown that abnormalities in the hippocampus as well as general atrophy of the brain can lead to dementia. Physicians are able to use these imaging tools in order to help determine the etiology of dementia. These types of imaging techniques can also be used in patients with DS in a similar manner. They can help to predict which patients are at a higher risk than others so that an intervention can be put in place earlier.

7. Practical applications

Physical activity of any kind will most likely improve cognitive functioning in persons with DS. Often physical activity that the person enjoys (e.g., dancing, gardening, and walking dog) are the types of programs that are sustained. Only 10–12% of people with DS learn to ride a bicycle and very few learn before 10 years old [52]. However, cycling does allow for fast rates of lower limb movement which is crucial because the increased movement rate may trigger the endogenous release of neurotrophic factors that facilitate the motoric and neural changes that underlie improved motor and cognitive function. To date, our stationary research bicycle is not for sale. One clinical research trial with Parkinson's patients used a tandem bicycle in which the front rider is typical and the back rider had Parkinson's disease. Because the pedals were yoked, the rear rider was pedaling at the same rate as the front rider. However, this may take a lot of practice to perform safely. An alternative recommendation is to be conscious of when you are physically active to try to increase the rate of movement whenever possible. For practical purposes, measure the rate of movement by counting the number of revolutions during a set time period (e.g., 10 s.) and extrapolating to one minute. Heart rate could be palpated or measured by a simple Polar HR monitor. In addition, Rate of Perceived Exertion should be monitored every five minutes especially in special populations such as DS where heart rate responses are different from those of the general population due to chronotropic incompetence [53]. The main goal is to have fun and be safe, and remember if you move faster, you may think faster!

Author details

Shannon D. R. Ringenbach*, Simon Holzapfel, Genna M. Mulvey and Sachin Pandya

*Address all correspondence to: Shannon.ringenbach@asu.edu

Arizona State University, Phoenix, AZ, USA

References

[1] National Down Syndrome Society. (2012). Down syndrome facts. Retrieved from http:// http://www.ndss.org/Down-Syndrome/Down-Syndrome-Facts/

[2] Lanfranchi, S., Jerman, O., Dal Pont, E., Alberti, A., & Vianello, R. (2010). Executive function in adolescents with Down syndrome. *Journal of Intellectual Disability Research, 54*(4), 308–319.

[3] Lezak, M. D. (1995). Neuropsychological Assessment. 3rd ed. Oxford University Press: New York.

[4] Das, J. P., Divis, B., Alexander J., Parrila R. K., & Naglieri, J. A. (1995). Cognitive decline due to aging among persons with Down syndrome. *Research in Developmental Disabilities, 16,* 461–478.

[5] Rowe, J., Lavender, A., & Turk, V. (2006). Cognitive executive function in Down's syndrome. *British Journal of Clinical Psychology, 45*(Pt 1), 5–17.

[6] Baddeley A. (2003). Working memory: Looking back and looking forward. *National Review of Neuroscience, 4,* 829–839.

[7] Maxwell, J. P., Masters, R. S. W., & Eves, F. F. (2003). The role of working memory in motor learning and performance. *Consciousness and Cognition, 12,* 376–402.

[8] Carney, D. P. J., Brown, J. H., & Henry, L. A. (2013). Executive function in Williams and Down syndrome. *Research in Developmental Disabilities, 34*(1), 46–55. doi: 10.1016/j.ridd.2012.07.013

[9] Lanfranchi, W., Cornoldi, C., & Vianello, R. (2004). Verbal and visuospatial working memory deficits in children with Down syndrome. *American Journal on Mental Retardation, 109,* 456–466.

[10] Frye, D., Zelazo, P. D., & Palfai, T. (1995). Theory of mind and rule-based reasoning. *Cognitive Development, 10,* 483–527.

[11] Davidson, M. C., Amso, D., Anderson, L. C., & Diamond, A. (2006). Development of cognitive control and executive functions from 4 to 13 years: Evidence from manipu-

lations of memory, inhibition, and task switching. Neuropsycholotgia, 44(11), 2037-2078.

[12] Periáñez, J.A., Maestú, F., Barceló F., Fernández, A., Amo, C., & Ortiz-Alonso, T. (2004). Spatiotemporal brain dynamics during preparatory set shifting. *Neuroimage, 21,* 687–695.

[13] Chapman, R. S. (2003). Language and communication in individuals with Down syndrome. In Abbeduto, L. (Ed). *International Review of Research in Mental Retardation: Language and Communication,* vol. 27. San Diego, CA, USA, Academic Press, pp. 1–34.

[14] Dykens, E. M., Hodapp, R. M., & Finucane, B. M. (2000). *Genetics and Mental Retardation Syndromes.* Paul H. Brookes: New York.

[15] Silverman, W. (2007). Down syndrome: cognitive phenotype. *Mental Retardation and Developmental Disabilities Research Reviews, 13,* 228–236.

[16] Baldo, J. V., Schwartz, S., Wilkins, D., & Dronkers, N. F. (2006). Role of frontal versus temporal cortex in verbal fluency as revealed by voxel-based lesion symptom mapping. *Journal oft he International Neuropsychological Society, 12,* 896–900. doi:10.1017/S1355617706061078.

[17] Nash, H. M. & Snowling, M. J. (2008). Semantic and phonological fluency in children with Down syndrome: Atypical organization of language or less efficient retrieval strategies? *Cognitive Neuropsychology, 25,* 690–703.

[18] Hillman, C. H., Erickson, K. I., & Kramer, A. F. (2008). Be smart, exercise your heart: Exercise effects on brain and cognition. *Nature Review Neuroscience,* 9(1), 58–65.

[19] Hillman, C. H., Snook, E. M., & Jerome, G.J. (2003). Acute cardiovascular exercise and executive control function. *International Journal of Psychophysiology,* 48(3), 307–314.

[20] Buck, S. M., Hillman, C. H., & Castelli, D. M. (2008). The relation of aerobic fitness to stroop task performance in preadolescent children. *Medicine in Science Sports and Exercise, 40*(1), 166–172.

[21] Hillman, C. H., Pontifex, M. B., Raine, L. B., Castelli, D. M., Hall, E. E., & Kramer, A. F. (2009). The effect of acute treadmill walking on cognitive control and academic achievement in preadolescent children. *Neuroscience, 159*(3), 1044–1054.

[22] Colcombe, S., & Kramer, A. F. (2003). Fitness effects on the cognitive function of older adults: A meta-analytic study. *Psychological Sciences, 14*(2), 125–130.

[23] van Uffelen, J. G., Chin, A. P. M. J., Hopman-Rock, M., & van Mechelen, W. (2008). The effects of exercise on cognition in older adults with and without cognitive decline: A systematic review. *Clinical Journal of Sport Medicine, 18,* 486–500.

[24] Llorens-Martín, M. V., Rueda, N., Tejeda, G. S., Flórez, J., Trejo, J. L., & Martínez-Cué, C. (2010). Effects of voluntary physical exercise on adult hippocampal neuro-

genesis and behavior of Ts65Dn mice, a model of Down syndrome. *Neuroscience, 171*(4): 1228–1240.

[25] Andriolo, R. B., El Dib, R. P., Ramos, L., Atallah, A. N., & da Silva, E.M. (2010). Aerobic exercise training programmes for improving physical and psychosocial health in adults with Down syndrome. *Cochrane Database Systems Review, 12*(5), CD005176.

[26] Latash, M. L. (1992). Motor control in Down syndrome: The role of adaptation and practice. *Journal of Developmental and Physical Disability, 4*, 227–261.

[27] Inui, N., Yamanishi, M., & Tada, S. (1985). Simple reaction times and timing of serial reactions of adolescents with mental retardation, autism, and Down syndrome. *Perceptual and Motor Skills, 81*(3 Pt 1), 739–745.

[28] Cioni, M., Cocilovo, A., Di Pasquale, F., Araujo, M. B., Siqueira, C. R., & Bianco, M. (1994). Strength deficit of knee extensor muscles of individuals with Down syndrome from childhood to adolescence. *American Journal of Mental Retardation, 99*(2), 166–174.

[29] Fernhall, B., Pitetti, K. H., Rimmer, J. H., & McCubbin, J. A. (1996). Cardiorespiratory capacity of individuals with mental retardation including Down syndrome. *Medicine and Science Sports and Exercise, 28*(3), 366–371.

[30] Barr, M., & Shields, N. (2011). Identifying the barriers and facilitators to participation in physical activity for children with Down syndrome. *Journal of Intellectual Disability Research, 55*(11), 1020–1033.

[31] Petzinger, G. M., Walsh, J. P., Akopian, G., Hogg, E., Abernathy, A., Arevalo, P., Turnquist, P., Vuckovic, M., Fisher, B. E., Togasaki, D. M., & Jakowec, M, W. (2007). Effects of treadmill exercise on dopaminergic transmission in the 1-methyl-4-phenyl-1, 2, 3, 6-tetrahydropyridine-lesioned mouse model of basal ganglia injury. *Journal of Neuroscience, 27*, 5291–5300.

[32] Ringenbach, S. D. R., Chen, C. C., Albert, A. R., Lichtsinn, K., & Alberts, J. L. (2013). Assisted cycle therapy (ACT): Implications for improvements in motor control. In Leitner, M. & Fuchs, M. (Eds.). *Motor Behavior and Control: New Research*, Hauppauge, NY: Nova Science Publishers Inc., pp. 103–114.

[33] Fisher, B. E., Petzinger, G. M., Nixon, K., Hogg, E., Bremmer, S., Meshul, C. K., Jakowec, M. W. (2004). Exercise-induced behavioral recovery and neuroplasticity in the 1-methyl-4-phenyl-1, 2, 3, 6-tetrahydropyridine- lesioned mouse basal ganglia. *Journal of Neurology Research, 77*, 378–390.

[34] Alberts, J. L., Linder, S. M., Penko, A. L., Lowe, M. J., & Phillips, M. (2011). It is not about the bike, it is about the pedaling: Forced exercise and Parkinson disease. *Exercise and Sport Science Review, 39*(4), 177–186.

[35] Ridgel, A. L., Vitek, J. L., & Alberts, J. L. (2009). Forced, not voluntary, exercise improves motor function in Parkinson's disease patients. *Neurorehabiltation and Neural Repair, 23*, 600–608.

[36] Fernhall, B. O., McCubbin, J. A., Pitetti, K. H., Rintala, P., Rimmer, J. H., Millar, A. L., & De Silva, A. (2001). Prediction of maximal heart rate in individuals with mental retardation. *Medicine and Science in Sports and Exercise, 33*(10), 1655–1660.

[37] American College of Sports Medicine. (2013). *ACSM's Guidelines for Exercise Testing and Prescription*. Baltimore, MD: Lippincott Williams & Wilkins.

[38] Dunn, D. M., & Dunn, L. M. (2007). *Peabody Picture Vocabulary Test—Fourth Edition*. San Antonio, TX: Pearson.

[39] Gabrieli, J. D., Poldrack, R. A., & Desmond, J. E. (1998). The role of left prefrontal cortex in language and memory. *Proceedings of the National Academy of Sciences, 95*(3), 906–913.

[40] Weiss, E. M., Siedentopf, C., Hofer, A., Deisenhammer, E. A., Hoptman, M. J., Kremser, C., Golaszewski, S., Felber, S., Fleischhacker, W. W., & Delazer, M. (2003). Brain activation pattern during a verbal fluency test in healthy male and female volunteers: A functional magnetic resonance imaging study. *Neuroscience Letters, 352*(3), 191–194.

[41] Fowler, A., Gelman, R., & Gleitman, L. R. (1994). The course of language learning in children with Down syndrome. *Constraints on language acquisition: Studies of atypical children*, 91–140.

[42] Hulme, C., & Mackenzie, S. (1992). *Working Memory and Severe Learning Difficulties*. Mahwah, NJ: Lawrence Erlbaum Associates, Inc.

[43] Pennington, B. F., Moon, J., Edgin, J., Stedron, J., & Nadel, L. (2003). The neuropsychology of Down syndrome: Evidence for hippocampal dysfunction. *Child development, 74*(1), 75–93.

[44] Iverson, G. L., & Franzen, M. D. (1994). The Recognition Memory Test, digit span, and Knox Cube Test as markers of malingered memory impairment. *Assessment, 1*(4), 323–334.

[45] Berman, K. F., Ostrem, J. L., Randolph, C., Gold, J., Goldberg, T. E., Coppola, R., Carson, R. E., Herscovitch, P., & Weinberger, D. R. (1995). Physiological activation of a cortical network during performance of the Wisconsin Card Sorting Test: A positron emission tomography study. *Neuropsychologia, 33*(8), 1027–1046.

[46] Nelson, H. E. (1976). A modified card sorting test sensitive to frontal lobe defects. *Cortex, 12*(4), 313–324.

[47] Cohen, J. 1988. Statistical power analysis for the behavioral sciences. Hillsdale, New Jersey: Lawrence Erlbaum Associates

[48] Miyake, A., Friedman, N. P., Emerson, M. J., Witzki, A. H., Howerter, A., & Wager, T. D. (2000). The unity and diversity of executive functions and their contributions to complex "frontal lobe" tasks: A latent variable analysis. *Cognitive Psychology, 41*(1), 49–100.

[49] Wisniewski, K. E., Wisniewski, H. M., & Wen, G. Y. (1985). Occurrence of neuropathological changes and dementia of Alzheimer's disease in Down's syndrome. *Annals of Neurology,* 17, 278–282.

[50] Hartley, D., Blumenthal, T., Carrillo, M., DiPaolo G., Esralew, L., Gardiner, K., Granholm, A. C., Igbal, K., Krams, M., Lemere, C., Lott, I., Mobley, W., Ness, S., Nixon, R., Potter, H., Reeves, R., Sabbagh, M., Silverman, W., Silverman, W., Tycko, B., Whitten, M., Wisniewski, T. (2014). Down syndrome and Alzheimer's disease: Common pathways, common goals. *Alzheimer's and Dementia,* 1–10. doi: 10.1016/j.jalz.2014.10.007. [Epub ahead of print]

[51] Zakzanis, K., Graham, S. J., & Campbell, Z. (2003). A meta-analysis of structural and functional brain imaging in dementia of the Alzheimer's type: A neuroimaging profile. *Neuropsychology Review, 13, 1-18.*(1).

[52] Ulrich, D. A., Burghardt, A. R., Lloyd, M., Tiernan, C., & Hornyak, J. E. (2011). Physical activity benefits of learning to ride a two-wheel bicycle for children with Down syndrome: A randomized trial. *Physical Therapy,* 91(10), 1463-1477.

[53] Baynard, T., Pitetti, K. H., Guerra, M., & Fernhall, B. (2004). Heart rate variability at rest and during exercise in persons with Down syndrome. Archives of Physical Medicine and Rehabilitation, 85(8), 1285–1290.

Section 3

Research Approaches on Down Syndrome

Chapter 5

Recent Advances in Research on Down Syndrome

Poulami Majumder, Pranami Bhaumik, Priyanka Ghosh, Mandar Bhattacharya, Sujoy Ghosh and Subrata Kumar Dey

Additional information is available at the end of the chapter

http://dx.doi.org/10.5772/60648

Abstract

Down syndrome (DS) or trisomy 21 is one of the most important genetic causes of mental retardation. Sincere and significant attempts have been made towards understanding the congenital diseases that affect DS patients. Better understanding of gene networks associated with such malformations will help to predict the complex genetic trait behind congenital disease in DS and will also provide the basis for tailored gene therapies that could begin to heal or prevent such malformation without the need to resort to invasive surgery. Further, susceptible mutation screening in women will also be helpful for both prenatal diagnosis of DS birth and assessing the risk of predisposition to Alzheimer's disease and congenital heart disease. Stress condition and neurodegeneration are two important markers in Down syndrome patients and mtDNA variation can also be used as an important biomarker. It has been suggested that nutraceuticals which reduce reactive oxygen species (ROS) level may be used to treat trisomy 21 condition. As mitochondria play a crucial role in the regulation of free radicals, only a detail analysis will reveal the origin of phenotypic characteristics among trisomy 21 DS patients. On the other hand, several mechanisms are responsible for neurodegeneration as well as altered cognition. It includes impaired neurogenesis leading to hypocellularity in the cortex, hippocampus and cerebellum, altered dendritic morphology, altered synapses, increased inhibition and neurodegeneration. The new knowledge of the pathogenic mechanisms in DS individuals has been acquired from mouse model. These studies provide the basis for developing new drugs for clinical trials in DS individuals and to sustain the hope that some of these drugs will be useful in treating intellectual disability in DS individuals.

Keywords: Down syndrome, trisomy 21, congenital heart disease, Alzheimer's disease, mitochondria, mouse model

1. Introduction

Down syndrome (DS) or trisomy 21 is the most frequent live born chromosomal aneuploidy in humans characterized by an extra chromosome 21 [1]. Myriad researches have contributed significantly towards understanding the management and control of disorders associated with Down syndrome. Since middle of 19th century, Down syndrome research has progressed alongside and in response to more general scientific advances. These researches attempt to cover the etiology, treatment, management, control, and prevention of DS. Both *in vitro* and *in vivo* experiments are carried out to understand the molecular mechanism of the origin of this aneuploidy. Many exciting areas are currently being investigated in relation to DS. A number of genes have been identified, which are putative candidates for phenotypic abnormalities. Use of Down syndrome mouse model, which is segmental trisomies of homologous segment of human chromosome 21, has facilitated greatly the process of reverse genetic approach to explore the gene–protein relationship in Down syndrome. Extensive studies are carried out in areas involving psycho-somatic and neural control of functions such as learning, behavior, and foetal brain development.

The research on Down syndrome has progressed and it can be assumed that people with Down syndrome will enjoy better quality of life in future. The most prevalent disorders among Down syndrome patients that have attracted the attention of research community are Alzheimer's disease and congenital heart defect. To go deep into the problem and to understand the exact etiology of these disorders, several approaches have been taken. One among them is mouse models for segmental trisomies, which are being used for better understanding of these disease conditions. The ultimate goal of all research approaches is to contribute toward the better management of lifestyle of Down syndrome individuals.

2. Congenital Heart Disease (CHD) in Down Syndrome

Down Syndrome (DS) is characterized by a combination of multifaceted congenital abnormalities with various degrees of severity. Among them cardiac anomalies are found in nearly 50% of DS cases.Cardiac abnormalities in DS include mainly atrioventricular septal defect (AVSD), ventricular septal defects (VSD), atrial septal defect(ASD) and few percentages of isolated tetralogy of fallot (TOF) of which approximately 40–60% includes an atrioventricular septal defect (AVSD) [2]. The developmental basis of atrioventricular septal defect also known as an atrioventricular canal defect or endocardial cushion defect is complex. This congenital cardiac anomaly occurs when the superior and inferior endocardial cushions fail to close completely, resulting in incomplete formation of atrial and ventricular valves and septa.. The tricuspid and mitral valves that normally separate the hearts upper and lower chambers are not formed as individual valves; instead, a single large valve is formed which does not close tightly. A large hole in the centre of the heart exists where the wall between the upper chambers join the wall between the lower chambers, allowing the blood to flow between all the chambers of the heart..This is called as a complete AVSD. In case of partial AVSD, there is usually a hole

http://dx.doi.org/10.5772/60648

in the wall between the atria or a hole in the wall between the ventricles near the middle of the heart, but there are usually two valves between the atria and ventricles and not a common valve as seen in complete AVSD. In partial AVSD, usually the mitral valve does not close completely and allows the blood to leak backward.

2.1. Recent studies on CHD

Higher incidence of congenital heart disease (CHD), especially AVSD, associated with DS has made the identification of CHD associated genes very challenging. Therefore, many researches focused on chromosome 21 (Ch21) genes, based on the hypothesis that overexpression of these genes may play a role in the etiology of AVSD in DS. Studies have implicated Ch21 genes, *COL6A1, COL6A2*, and *DSCAM* as potential contributors to heart defects in DS [3–5]. A recent study has shown that overexpression of *DSCAM* and *COL6A2* cooperatively causes atrial defects in mice [6]. Recently a candidate gene approach carried out among Down syndrome individuals with AVSD and Down syndrome without CHD suggests a potential contribution of VEGF-A, ciliome, hedgehog and folate pathway genes such as *MTHFR, MTRR, SLC19A1, MTR*, and *CBS* to the pathogenesis of CHD in DS [7–9].

Many studies based on the premise that myriad of genes are involved in cardiogenesis, and perturbation in any of this gene by mutation can cause CHD, therefore, highlighting the role of non-chromosome 21 gene mutation to play a key role in the etiology of AVSD in DS. For example, pathogenic mutations in the CRELD1 gene have been found to be associated with AVSD [10]. Studies have also shown that how polymorphic haplotypes of CRELD1 increase the risk of AVSD, and the susceptibility is exacerbated in DS, possibly due to the trisomy 21 genetic background [11]. Furthermore, there is a growing body of evidence, highlighting the role of epigenetic in the development of AVSD in DS [12].

There are multiple risk alleles that play an important role in the pathogenesis of congenital heart disease (CHD) in DS. Alone trisomy 21 background is not enough to reach the threshold needed for the development of CHD. There exists a multifactorial model where genetic and epigenetic variants, unknown environmental factors, and stochastic events are required in addition to trisomy 21 background to cross the threshold for developing CHD in DS.

3. Relationship between Alzheimer's Disease and Down Syndrome

Alzheimer's disease (AD) is well known as the major cause of dementia in elderly people, characterized mainly by cognitive decline and other motor dysfunction. Several lines of researches indicate that Alzheimer's disease share some common genetic factors with Down syndrome. Imaging techniques have confirmed AD-like pathogenic signs in the brain of most DS patients after 40 years of age [13, 14]. Frequent birth of babies with DS is evident in families with AD patients. Moreover, greater number of AD patients are counted among the relatives of DS. Neurons progressively and irreversibly die chiefly due to deposition of amyloid beta protein and eventually perturb neurosynaptic circuits in the brain [15]. The amyloid hypothesis states that APP (amyloid precursor protein) gene, located on chromosome 21, encodes for amyloid precursor protein which is proteolyzed by enzymatic cascade and eventually produce amyloid beta protein that in turn oligomerizes and forms beta-plaque [16]. The increased amyloid load due to overexpression of APP in trisomy 21 cells is hypothesized to be a cause of AD in DS [17]. Moreover, APP gene mutations are also found in both AD and DS [18]. Apolipoprotein E (APOE) is one of the key genes involved in the manifestation in sporadic AD cases; epsilon 4 allele of this gene is reported to be associated with deterioration in cognitive ability in DS patients [19].

3.1. Theory of chromosomal missegregation

Scientists have pointed out that chromosomal segregation error may be the possible underlying molecular link between these two disorders [20, 21]. Abnormality in cell cycle regulation due to mutations in different genes involved in both sporadic and familial AD cases is also apparent [20, 22, 23]. According to this theory, AD patients bear mosaic aneuploid cells in central and peripheral nervous system which are susceptible to apoptosis [20]. Besides neurons and buccal cells, lymphocytes are also found to be trisomic for chromosome 21 [23–27]. Again, inflammatory responses induced by overexpression of IL-1 in trisomic microglia increase amyloid beta production [28].

3.2. Relationship between Alzheimer's Disease and mothers of Down Syndrome child

Researches revealed that women giving birth to Down syndrome (DS) babies at younger age are prone to have AD with aging [29]. Young mothers bearing DS offspring are also found to possess APOE epsilon 4 allele with a higher frequency [30]. Presenilin 1(PSEN-1) is another important gene playing a role in AD pathogenesis. Trisomy 21 aneuploidy and chromosomal instability are evident in AD patients with mutation in PSEN-1 gene [20, 31]. Association of polymorphism of PSEN-1 gene (rs165932) is also established in young mother, giving birth to DS babies due to nondisjunction error in second meiotic division of oocyte [32]. It is postulated that accumulation of mosaic trisomy 21 cells in both somatic and germline tissue make those women prone to AD in their later life and also responsible for giving birth to DS child. Thus the theory of chromosomal missegregation offers us a new insight into the understanding the molecular mechanism that bridges Down syndrome with Alzheimer's disease.

3.3. Other common factors linking Alzheimer's Disease and Down Syndrome

3.3.1. Mitochondrial dysfunction

Mitochondrial dysfunction is associated with AD pathology [33]. Protein members of mitochondrial electron transport chain are found malfunctioning in Alzheimer's disease [34]. Diminished cytochrome oxidase activity reflecting improper functioning of mitochondria in AD patients is revealed by biochemical, histochemical, and immune-histochemical analysis [35]. Showing similarity with AD cases, dysregulation in mitochondria is evident in Down syndrome etiology [36]. Individuals with DS also exhibit reduced activity of several mitochondrial enzymes, including cytochrome oxidase [37]. Thus oxidative stress due to mitochondrial dysfunction is typical in both AD and DS.

http://dx.doi.org/10.5772/60648

3.3.2. *Abnormal tau phosphorylation*

Another very strong hallmark of AD is the presence of intra-neuronal neurofibrillary tangle made up of hyperphosphorylated tau protein. The neurotoxic effect of these tangles makes the neurons vulnerable to death. Researchers revealed that the abnormality in tau phosphorylation is seen both in AD and DS [38]. A kinase enzyme called "dual-specificity tyrosine phosphorylated and regulated kinase 1A" or DYRK1A phosphorylates tau protein. This gene is mapped in the Down syndrome critical region of chromosome 21, hence present in triple copies in DS patients, giving rise to enhanced production of DYRK1A [39]. Moreover, hippocampal, neocortical, and entorhinal-cortical neurons show increased DYRK1A immune-reactivity in both AD and DS patients [40].

3.3.3. *Altered endocytic pathway activity*

Altered endocytic pathway activity is another common phenomenon that bridges both disorders [41]. Neurons internalize and modify extracellular molecules from cell surface via endocytosis and relay signals for intracellular biosynthetic pathways to occur. Initial processing of APP and APOE proteins and cellular uptake of amyloid beta take place in the early endosomes. Bigger size of early endosomes was seen in AD brain, suggesting increased endocytic pathway activity [42, 43]. Several growth factors, cell surface receptors, and other plasma proteins can be erroneously degraded and processed by activated early endosome in neurons, exposing them in peril. Such improper endolysis of neuronal glucose transporter is found responsible in reduced uptake of glucose in AD brain [44, 45]. Strikingly, pyramidal neurons with enlarged early endosomes are also found in DS fetus at 28 weeks of gestation [41].

4. Mitochondrial DNA analysis in Down Syndrome patients

The double-stranded circular mammalian mtDNA molecule of 16.5 kb contains a single long noncoding region, a displacement loop (D loop) region, the promoters for transcription of both mtDNA strands and the origin of leading strand replication (O_H). The origin of lagging strand replication (O_L) is surrounded in a cluster of tRNA genes. mtDNA codes two rRNAs (12S and 16S rRNA), 13 mRNAs (ND1–6, ND4L, Cyt b, COI–III, ATP6, and ATP8), and 22 tRNAs (F, V, L1, I, M, W, D, K, G, R, H, S1, L2, T, P, E, S2, Y, C, N, A, and Q).

4.1. Why study mitochondria in Down Syndrome patients?

Mitochondria controls one of the most important biochemical pathways, oxidative phosphorylation (OXPHOS). A mild imbalance in mitochondrial function or a slight change in mitochondrial structural integrity might lead to a severe cellular oxidative damage and finally apoptosis. As Down syndrome is an AD-like disease condition, oxidative stress plays a key role in disease pathogenesis with inevitable involvement of mitochondria.

4.2. Structural and biochemical anomalies in mitochondria among Down Syndrome patients

Several mitochondrial anomalies have been reported in trisomy 21 patients over the years of research. Decreased levels of several mitochondrial enzymes such as monoamine oxidase, cytochrome oxidase, and isocitrate dehydrogenase have been observed in trisomy 21 patients [37]. At genetic level, downregulation of mitochondrial enzyme genes and upregulation of mitochondrial extracellular matrix protein genes have been found out by oligonucleotide microarray in Down syndrome fetus [46]. The level of another important enzyme, pyruvate dehydrogenase, is found to decrease in the brain of trisomy 16 mouse [47–49]. At structural level, heavy accumulation of microfilaments, tubules, and abnormally shaped mitochondria is reported in cerebellar neuron of trisomy 16 mice [50]. The 20 kD complex has also been found out to be downregulated [49]. Mitochondrial membrane potential in peripheral blood mononuclear cell (PBMC) is decreased among Down syndrome individuals, which indicates severe impairment of mitochondrial function [51].

4.3. mtDNA variations among Down Syndrome patients

mtDNA because of its close proximity to mitochondrial membrane might undergo severe changes due to reactive oxygen species (ROS). mtDNA contains hyper variable D-loop region (HDR) and semi-variable regulatory control region (RCR). This particular region is responsible for overall mtDNA transcription mechanism and any adverse change in this region hampers the overall transcriptional procedure. Several heteroplasmic mutations have been observed in Down syndrome brains which include G70A, C114T, C150T, G185A, and 309.1-3insC. Down syndrome lymphoblasts and control lymphoblast share the A73G variant while they more commonly have the 309.1inC, A357G, and 522–523delCA [52].

5. Mouse model

In recent years, mouse models are used as standard tool for *in vivo* study. It provides an insight into the normal functions and regulation of genes and how these are altered in disease and how they contribute to severity of this disease. Administration of certain drugs as well as information on drug action, efficacy, and side effects also can be evaluated by this animal model [53]. So mouse models are used to enhance our knowledge on human genes, their functions, interactions, and biochemistry. The most studied mouse model for DS is the Ts65Dn mouse which possesses an extra copy of the chromosome number 16. The distal segment of mouse chromosome 16 (MMU16) is homologous to nearly the entire long arm of human chromosome 21 (HSA21), and thus trisomic mouse models are developed in such a way that it genetically resembles human condition. Ts65Dn and Ts1Cje mice mimic many of the behavioral, learning, and developmental deficits characteristics in DS individuals [54–58]. The availability of sophisticated tools for mouse genetics and the conserved synteny between MMU16 and HSA21 have provided the basis for the development of many mouse models of DS. This similarity allows to test the critical region concept and to perform a genetic dissection of the complex DS phenotype.. The knowledge obtained from these models about the neurobiology of DS have yielded the development and analysis of several therapeutic strategies that could potentially be used to attenuate cognitive impairments in DS individuals. s

5.1. Recent studies on mouse model

Mouse modeling is a very useful technique to understand the neural mechanism underlying the cognitive impairment seen in Down syndrome. The association of Alzheimer's disease with Down syndrome and the regulation of involved genes are being investigated via mouse model [59]. DS individuals typically display an average Intelligence Quotient (IQ) of 50 (ranging from 30 to 70) and show an array of altered cognitive and behavioral phenotypes, including the incomplete and delayed acquisition of motor, linguistic, and visual-spatial abilities, impairments in learning and memory, and neurobehavioral disorders [60–62]. Holtzman et al. (1996) suggest that Ts65Dn mice are the most useful animal model to study the developmental and degenerative abnormalities in the DS brain *in vivo* [56]. Studies show that Ts65Dn mice mimic the specific age-related decrease in cholinergic function seen in Down syndrome and Alzheimer's disease [63]. The degeneration of cholinergic neurons in basal forebrain is age related and this finding raises the possibility that this model may be used further to understand mechanisms underlying selective neuronal vulnerability seen in DS and AD. Ts65Dn mice also carry a trisomy of MMU17 containing 60 genes nonhomologous to Hsa21, so this model does not have perfect construct validity [64]. Mouse modeling also revealed that the nerve growth factor (NGF) is required for the normal differentiation of basal forebrain cholinergic neurons (BFCNs) and the abnormalities in NGF levels or signaling in Ts65Dn mice may determine the regulating factors in neuronal degeneration [64]. GABA (gamma amino butyric acid) is an important neurotransmitter that regulates neuronal proliferation, migration, differentiation, and integration of newly generated neurons [65]. It has been suggested that upregulation of presynaptic GABA may be responsible for the increased hippocampal inhibitory postsynaptic potentials (IPSPs) observed in these mice [66]. Netzer et al. have tested the effect of β-amyloid reductions in the Ts65Dn mice which altered its phenotypes [67]. They administered the gamma secretase inhibitor DAPT (*N*-[*N*-(3,5-difluorophenacetyl)-L-alanyl]-*S*-phenylglycine *t*-butyl ester) into mice and this treatment reduced β-amyloid levels and rescued spatial learning in these mice. β-amyloid is a regulator of the glutamatergic system, and the authors proposed that the cognitive enhancing effects of DAPT could be mediated by an enhancement and/or a regulation of excitatory synaptic transmission. It has been proposed that pharmacological enhancements of the cholinergic system help to diminish the cognitive deterioration in DS with AD. Another research revealed that an acetylcholinesterase inhibitor, Donepezil, is widely prescribed to enhance cholinergic transmission to treat DS with dementia. However, the chronic administration of Donepezil did not improve learning and memory in Ts65Dn mice and causes ambiguous results in young adult individuals with DS [68]. Another drug named piracetam shows cognitive-enhancing effects in patients with a number of cognitive disorders and dementia and also in mouse models though the mechanisms underlying these effects are unknown [69]. However, piracetam treatment did not improve cognitive impairments in children with DS or in the Ts65Dn mouse [70].

The first partial trisomic models, the Ts65Dn and Ts1Cje models, demonstrated that DS phenotypes could be recapitulated in mice. More recently, knock-out and transgenic mice are developed in different laboratories for particular genes, though there is no mouse model that perfectly mimics a human condition. In the last 20 years, mouse models, particularly the Ts65Dn mouse, have been widely used to understand the neurobiological basis of intellectual disability.

Acknowledgements

We are thankful to Indian Council of Medical Research (ICMR), New Delhi, for granting us a project on Down syndrome and also for financial assistance.

Author details

Poulami Majumder[1], Pranami Bhaumik[1], Priyanka Ghosh[1], Mandar Bhattacharya[1], Sujoy Ghosh[2] and Subrata Kumar Dey[1*]

*Address all correspondence to: subratadey184@gmail.com

1 Department of Biotechnology, West Bengal University of Technology, Salt Lake, Sector I, Kolkata, West Bengal, India

2 Department of Zoology, University of Calcutta, Ballygunge Science College Campus, Kolkata, West Bengal, India

Authors declare no conflict of interest.

References

[1] Patterson D. (2009), "Molecular genetic analysis of Down syndrome," Human Genet. 126(1): 195–214.

[2] Freeman S. B., Taft L. F., Dooley K. J., Allran K., Sherman S. L., Hassold T. J., Khoury M. J., Saker D. M. (1998), "Population-based study of congenital heart defects in Down syndrome," Am J Med.Genet. 80: 213–217.

[3] Davies G. E., Howard C. M., Farrer M. J., Coleman M. M., Cullen L. M.,Williamson R., Wyse R. K. H., Kessling A. M. (1994), "Unusual genotypes in the COL6A1 gene in parents of children with trisomy-21 and major congenital heart defects," Hum Genet. 93: 443–446.

[4] Klewer S. E., Krob S. L., Kolker S. J., Kitten G. T. (1998), "Expression of type VI collagen in the developing mouse heart," Dev Dyn. 211: 248–255.

[5] Barlow G. M., Chen X. N., Shi Z. Y., Lyons G. E., Kurnit D. M., Celle L.,Spinner N. B., Zackai E., Pettenati M. J., Van Riper A. J., Vekemans M. J., Mjaatvedt C. H., Korenberg J. R. (2001), "Down syndrome congenital heart disease: a narrowed region and a candidate gene," Genet Med. 3: 91–101.

[6] GrossmanT. R., Gamliel A., Wessells R. J., Taghli-Lamallem O., Jepsen K., Ocorr K., Korenberg J. R., Peterson K. L., Rosenfeld M. G., Bodmer R., Bier E. (2001), "Overexpression of DSCAM and COL6A2 cooperatively generates congenital heart defects," PLoS Genet. 7:e1002344.

[7] Ackerman C., Locke A. E., Fiengold E., Reshey B., Espana K., Thusberg J., Mooney S., Bean L. J., Dooley K. J., Cua C. L. et al.(2012), "An excess of deleterious variants in VEGF-A pathway genes in Down-syndrome-associated atrioventricularseptal defects," Am J Med.Genet. 91(4): 646–659.

[8] Ripoll C., Rivals I., Ait Yahya-Graison E., Dauphinot L., Paly E., Mircher C., Ravel A., Grattau Y., Blehautt H., Megarbane A. et al. (2012), "Molecular signatures of cardiac defects in Down syndrome lymphoblastoid cell lines suggest altered ciliome and Hedgehog pathways," PLoS One. 7(8): e41616.

[9] Locke A. E., Dooley K. J.,Tinker S. W., Cheong S. Y., Feingold E., Allen E. G., Freeman S. B., Torfs C. P., Cua C. L., Epstein M. P., Wu M. C., Lin X., Capone G., Sherman S. L., Bean L. J. (2010), "Variation in folate pathway genes contributes to risk of congenital heart defects among individuals with Down syndrome genetic," Epidemiology. 34: 613–623.

[10] Robinson S. W., Morris C. D., Goldmuntz E., Reller M. D., Jones M. A., Steiner R. D., Maslen C. L. (2003), "Missense mutations in CRELD1 are associated with cardiac atrioventricularseptal defects," Am J Hum Genet. 72: 1047–1052.

[11] Ghosh P., Bhaumik P., Ghosh S., Ozbek U., Feingold E., Maslen C., Sarkar B., Pramanik V., Biswas P., Bandyopadhyay B., Dey S. K. (2012), "Polymorphic haplotype of CRELD1 differentially predispose Down syndrome and euploids individuals to atrioventricularseptal defect," Am J Med Genet Part A. 158A: 2843–2848.

[12] Chowdhury S., Erickson S. W., MacLeod S. L., Cleves M. A., Hu P., Karim M. A., Hobbs C. A. (2011), "Maternal genome-wide DNA methylation patterns and congenital heart defects," Plos One 6(1):e16506.

[13] Mann D. M., Esiri M. M. (1989), "The pattern of acquisition of plaques and tangles in the brains of patients under 50 years of age with Down's syndrome," J Neurol Sci. 89: 169–179.

[14] Cork L. C. (1990), "Neuropathology of Down syndrome and Alzheimer disease," Am J Med Genet. Suppl 7: 282–286.

[15] Yatham L. N., McHale P. A., Kinsella A. (1988), "Down syndrome and its association with Alzheimer's disease," Acta Psychiatr Scand. 77: 38–41.

[16] Hardy J. A., Higgins G. A. (1992), "Alzheimer's disease: the amyloid cascade hypothesis," Science. 256(5054): 184–185.

[17] Rumble B., Retallack R., Hilbich C., Simms G., Multhaup G., Martins R., Hockey A., Montgomery P., Beyreuther K., Masters C. L. (1989), "Amyloid A4 protein and its precursor in Down's syndrome and Alzheimer's disease," N Engl J Med. 320(22): 1446–1452.

[18] van Leeuwen F. W., de Kleijn D. P., van den Hurk H. H., Neubauer A., Sonnemans M. A., Sluijs J. A., Köycü S., Ramdjielal R. D., Salehi A., Martens G. J., Grosveld F. G., Peter J., Burbach H., Hol E. M. (1998), "Frameshift mutants of beta amyloid precursor protein and ubiquitin-B in Alzheimer's and Down patients," Science. 279(5348): 242–247.

[19] Del Bo R., Comi G. P., Bresolin N., Castelli E., Conti E., Degiuli A., Ausenda C. D., Scarlato G. (1997), "The apolipoprotein E epsilon4 allele causes a faster decline of cognitive performances in Down's syndrome subjects," J Neurol Sci. 145(1): 87–91.

[20] Potter H. (1991), "Review and hypothesis: Alzheimer disease and Down syndrome chromosome 21 nondisjunction may underlie both disorders," Am J Hum Genet. 48: 1192–1200.

[21] Potter H., Wefes I. M., Nilsson L. N. (2001), "The inflammation-induced pathological chaperones ACT and apo-E are necessary catalysts of Alzheimer amyloid formation," Neurobiol Aging. 22(6): 923–930.

[22] Arendt T., Rodel L., Gartner U., Holzer M. (1996), "Expression of the cyclin-dependent kinase inhibitor p16 in Alzheimer's disease," Neuroreports. 7(18): 3047–3049.

[23] Yang Y., Geldmacher D. S., Herrup K. (2001), "DNA replication precedes neuronal cell death in Alzheimer's disease," J Neurosci. 21(8): 2661–2668.

[24] Mosch B., Morawski M., Mittag A., Lenz D., Tarnok A., Arendt T. (2007), "Aneuploidy and DNA replication in the normal human brain and Alzheimer's disease," J Neurosci. 27(26): 6859–6867.

[25] Thomas P., Fenech M. (2008), "Chromosome 17 and 21 aneuploidy in buccal cells is increased with ageing and in Alzheimer's disease," Mutagenesis. 23(1): 57–65.

[26] Migliore L., Botto N., Scarpato R., Petrozzi L., Cipriani G., Bonuccelli U. (1999), "Preferential occurrence of chromosome 21 malsegregation in peripheral blood lymphocytes of Alzheimer disease patients," Cytogenet Cell Genet. 87(1–2): 41–46.

[27] Trippi F., Botto N., Scarpato R., Petrozzi L., Bonuccelli U., Latorraca S., Sorbi S., Migliore L. (2001), "Spontaneous and induced chromosome damage in somatic cells of sporadic and familial Alzheimer's disease patients," Mutagenesis. 16(4): 323–327.

[28] Potter H. (2008), "Down syndrome and Alzheimer's disease: two sides of the same coin," Future Neurology. 3: 29–37.

[29] Schupf N., Kapell D., Nightingale B., Lee J. H., Mohlenhoff J., Bewley S., Ottman R., Mayeux R. (2001), "Specificity of the fivefold increase in AD in mothers of adults with Down syndrome," Neurology. 57: 979–984.

[30] Avramopoulos D., Mikkelsen M., Vassilopoulos D., Grigoriadou M., Petersen M. B. (1996), "Apolipoprotein E allele distribution in parents of Down's syndrome children," Lancet. 347(9005): 862–865.

[31] Geller L. N., Potter H. (1999), "Chromosome missegregation and trisomy 21 mosaicism in Alzheimer's disease," Neurobiol Dis. 6(3): 167–179.

[32] Petersen M. B., Karadima G., Samaritaki M., Avramopoulos D., Vassilopoulos D., Mikkelsen M. (2000), "Association between presenilin-1 polymorphism and maternal meiosis II errors in Down syndrome," Am J Med Genet. 93: 366–372.

[33] Hauptmann S., Keil U., Scherping I., Bonert A., Eckert A., Müller W. E. (2006), "Mitochondrial dysfunction in sporadic and genetic Alzheimer's disease," Exp Gerontol. 41(7): 668–673.

[34] Blass J. P, Baker A. C., Ko L., Black R. S. (1990), "Induction of Alzheimer antigens by an uncoupler of oxidative phosphorylation," Arch Neurol. 47: 864–869.

[35] Wong-Riley M., Antuono P., Ho K.V., Egan R., Hevner R., Liebl W., Huang Z., Rachel R., Jones J. (1997), "Cytochrome oxidase in Alzheimer's disease: biochemical, histochemical, and immunohistochemical analyses of the visual and other system," Vision Res. 37: 3593–3608.

[36] Pagano G., Castello G. (2012), "Oxidative stress and mitochondrial dysfunction in Down syndrome," Adv Exp Med Biol. 724: 291–299.

[37] Prince J, Jia S, Båve U, Annerén G, Oreland L. (1994), Mitochondrial enzyme deficiencies in Down's syndrome. J Neural Transm Park Dis Dement Sect. 8(3): 171–181. PubMed PMID: 7748461.

[38] Nichols T. W. (2014), "Hyperphosphorylation of Tau Protein in Down's dementia and Alzheimer's disease: methylation and implications in prevention and therapy," J Alzheimers Dis Parkinsonism. 4: 5.

[39] Wegiel J., Kaczmarski W., Barua M., Kuchna I , Nowicki K., Wang K. C. (2011), "Link between DYRK1A over expression and several-fold enhancement of neurofibrillary degeneration with 3-repeat tau protein in Down syndrome," J Neuropathol Exp Neurol. 70: 36–50.

[40] Ferrer I., Barrachina M., Puig B., Martínez de Lagrán M., Martí E., Avila J., Dierssen M. (2005), "Constitutive Dyrk1A is abnormally expressed in Alzheimer disease,

Down syndrome, Pick disease, and related transgenic models," Neurobiol Dis. 20(2): 392–400.

[41] Cataldo A. M., Peterhoff C. M., Troncoso J. C., Gomez-Isla T., Hyman B. T., Nixon R. A. (2000), "Endocytic pathway abnormalities precede amyloid beta deposition in sporadic Alzheimer's disease and Down syndrome: differential effects of APOE genotype and presenilin mutations," Am J Pathol. 157(1): 277–286.

[42] Gorvel J. P., Chavrier P., Zerial M., Gruenberg J. (1991), "Rab5 controls early endosome fusion in vitro," Cell. 64: 915–925.

[43] Bucci C, Parton R. G., Mather I. H., Stunnenberg H., Simons K., Hoflack B., Zerial M. (1992), "The small GTPase rab5 functions as a regulatory factor in the early endocytic pathway". Cell. 70: 715–728.

[44] Simpson I. A., Chundu KR, Davies-Hill T, Honer WG, Davies P. (1994), "Decreased concentrations of GLUT1 and GLUT3 glucose transporters in the brains of patients with Alzheimer's disease," Ann Neurol. 35: 546–551.

[45] Vannucci S. J., Reinhart R., Maher F., Bondy C. A., Lee W. H., Vannucci R. C., Simpson I. A. (1998), "Alterations in GLUT1 and GLUT3 glucose transporter gene expression following unilateral hypoxia-ischemia in the immature rat brain," Brain Res Dev Brain Res. 107: 255–264.

[46] Conti A., Fabbrini F., D'Agostino P., Negri R., Greco D., Genesio R., D'Armiento M., Olla C., Paladini D., Zannini M., Nitsch L. (2007), "Altered expression of mitochondrial and extracellular matrix genes in the heart of human fetuses with chromosome 21 trisomy," BMC Genomics. 8: 268. PubMed PMID: 17683628; PubMed Central PMCID: PMC1964766.

[47] Schuchmann S., Heinemann U. (2000), "Increased mitochondrial superoxide generation in neurons from trisomy 16 mice: a model of Down's syndrome," Free Radic Biol Med. 28(2): 235–250.

[48] Capone G., Kim P., Jovanovich S., Payne L., Freund L., Welch K., Miller E., Trush M. (2002), "Evidence for increased mitochondrial superoxide production in Down syndrome," Life Sci.70(24): 2885–2995.

[49] Bambrick L. L., Fiskum G. (2007), "Mitochondrial dysfunction in mouse trisomy 16 brain," Brain Res. 2008 Jan 10;1188: 9–16. Epub. PubMed PMID: 18061151.

[50] Bersu E. T., Ahmad F. J., Schwei M. J., et al. (1998), "Cytoplasmic abnormalities in cultured cerebellar neurons from the trisomy 16 mouse," Brain Res Dev Brain Res. 109: 115–120.

[51] Roat E., Prada N., Ferraresi R., et al (2007). Mitochondrial alterations and tendency to apoptosis in peripheral blood cells from children with Down syndrome. FEBS Lett; 581: 521–525.

[52] Coskun P. E., Wyrembak J., Derbereva O., Melkonian G., Doran E., Lott I. T., Head E., Cotman C. W., Wallace D. C. (2010), "Systemic mitochondrial dysfunction and the etiology of Alzheimer's disease and down syndrome dementia," J Alzheimers Dis. 20 Suppl2:S293–310. doi: 10.3233/JAD-2010-100351.

[53] Das I., Reeves R. H. (2011), "The use of mouse models to understand and improve cognitive deficits in Down syndrome," Disease Models & Mechanisms. 4: 596–606.

[54] Galdzicki Z., Siarey R., Pearce R., Stoll J., Rapoport S. I. (2001), "On the cause of mental retardation in Down syndrome: extrapolation from full and segmental trisomy 16 mouse models," Brain Res Brain Res Rev. 35: 115–145.

[55] Galdzicki Z., Siarey R. J. (2003), "Understanding mental retardation in Down's syndrome using trisomy 16 mouse models," Genes Brain Behav. 2: 167–178.

[56] Holtzman D. M., Santucci D., Kilbridge J., Couzens J. C., Daniels S. E., Johnson R. M., Chen K., Fontana D. J., Sun Y., Carlson E., Alleva E., Epstein C. J., Mobley W.C. (1996), "Developmental abnormalities and age-related neurodegeneration in a mouse model of Down syndrome," Proc. Natl. Acad. Sci. USA. 93: 13333–13338.

[57] Reeves R. H., Irving N. G., Moran T. H., Wohn A., Kitt C., Sisodia S. S., Schmidt C., Bronson R. T., Davisson M. T. (1995), "A mouse model for Down syndrome exhibits learning and behavior deficits," Nat Genet. 11: 177–184.

[58] Sago H., Carlson E. J., Smith D. J., Kilbridge J., Rubin E. M., Mobley W. C., Epstein C. J., Huang T. T. (1998), "Ts1Cje, a partial trisomy 16 mouse model for Down syndrome, exhibits learning and behavioral abnormalities," Proc Natl Acad Sci USA. 95: 6256–6261.

[59] Cenini G., Dowling A. L. S., Beckett T. L., Barone E., Mancuso C., Murphy M. P., et al. (2012), "Association between frontal cortex oxidative damage and beta-amyloid as a function of age in Down syndrome," Biochimica et Biophysica Acta. 1822(2): 130–138.

[60] Vicari S. (2006), "Motor development and neuropsychological patterns in persons with Down syndrome," Behavior Genetics. 36 (3): 355–364.

[61] Chapman R.S., Hesketh L. J. (2000), "Behavioral phenotype of individuals with down syndrome," Mental Retardation and Developmental Disabilities Research Reviews. 6(2): 84–95.

[62] Nadel L. (2003), "Down's syndrome: a genetic disorder in biobehavioral perspective," Genes Brain and Behavior. 2(3): 156–166.

[63] Kish S., Karlinsky H., Becker L., Gilbert J., Rebbetoy M., Chang L. J., DiStefano L., Hornykiewicz O., Ritchie I. M., Urquhart, A. (1989), "Down's syndrome individuals begin life with normal levels of brain cholinergic markers," J Neurochem. 52(4): 1183–1187.

[64] Duchon A., Raveau M., Chevalier C., Nalesso V., Sharp A.J., Herault Y. (2011), "Identification of the translocation breakpoints in the Ts65Dn and Ts1Cje mouse lines: relevance for modeling Down syndrome," Mammalian Genome. 22(11–12): 674–684.

[65] Ge S., Goh E. L. K., Sailor K. A, Kitabatake Y., Ming G. L., Song H. (2006), "GABA regulates synaptic integration of newly generated neurons in the adult brain," Nature. 439(7076): 589–593.

[66] Kleschevnikov A. M., Belichenko P. V., Gall J., George L., Nosheny R, Maloney M. T., Salehi A., Mobley W. C. (2012), "Increased efficiency of the $GABA_A$ and $GABA_B$ receptor-mediated neurotransmission in the Ts65Dn mouse model of Down syndrome," Neurobiology of Disease. 45(2): 683–691.

[67] Netzer W. J., Powell C., Nong Y., Blundell J., Wong L., Duff K., Flajolet M., Greengard P. (2010), "Lowering beta-amyloid levels rescues learning and memory in a Down syndrome mouse model," PLoS One. 5(6): e10943.

[68] Rueda N., Florez J., Martinez-Cue C. (2008), "Chronic pentylenetetrazole but not donepezil treatment rescues spatial cognition in Ts65Dn mice, a model for Down syndrome," Neuroscience Letters. 433: 22–27.

[69] Lobaugh N. J., Karaskov V., Tombough V. Rombough V., Rovet J., Bryson S., Greenbaum R. et al. (2001), "Piracetam therapy does not enhance cognitive function in children with Down syndrome," Archives of Pediatrics & Adolescent Medicine, 155: 442–448.

[70] Moran T. H., Capone G. T., Knipp S., Davisson M. T., Reeves R. H., Gearhart J. D. (2002), "The effects of piracetam on cognitive performance in a mouse model of Down's syndrome," Physiology & Behavior. 77: 403–409.

Chapter 6

Double Aneuploidy in Down Syndrome

Fatma Soylemez

Additional information is available at the end of the chapter

http://dx.doi.org/10.5772/60438

Abstract

Aneuploidy is the second most important category of chromosome mutations relating to abnormal chromosome number. It generally arises by nondisjunction at either the first or second meiotic division. However, the existence of two chromosomal abnormalities involving both autosomal and sex chromosomes in the same individual is relatively a rare phenomenon. The underlying mechanism involved in the formation of double aneuploidy is not well understood. Parental origin is studied only in a small number of cases and both nondisjunctions occurring in a single parent is an extremely rare event. This chapter reviews the characteristics of double aneuploidies in Down syndrome have been discussed in the light of the published reports.

Keywords: Double aneuploidy, Down Syndrome, Klinefelter Syndrome, Chromosome abnormalities

1. Introduction

With the discovery in 1956 that the correct chromosome number in humans is 46, the new area of clinical cytogenetic began its rapid growth. Several major chromosomal syndromes with altered numbers of chromosomes were reported, such as Down syndrome (trisomy 21), Turner syndrome (45,X) and Klinefelter syndrome (47,XXY). Since then it has been well established that chromosome abnormalities contribute significantly to genetic disease resulting in reproductive loss, infertility, stillbirths, congenital anomalies, abnormal sexual development, mental retardation and pathogenesis of malignancy [1]. Clinical features of patients with common autosomal or sex chromosome aneuploidy is shown in Table 1.

Trisomy 21 or Down syndrome is one of the best-recognized and most common chromosome disorders caused by the presence of all or part of a third copy of chromosome 21 (Figure 1). It is the single most common genetic cause for mental retardation. The incidence of Down syndrome is approximately 1/800 newborns [2]. The risk for having a child with Down syndrome increases with maternal age. Clinical features include mental and growth retardation, characteristic faces and other abnormalities described in Table 1. Approximately 94% of Down syndrome patients have trisomy 21 resulting from meiotic nondisjunction, the failure of homologous chromosomes or sister chromatids to separate during cell division. The generally exponential increase in the frequency of nondisjunction with increasing maternal age is correlated with a decline in genetic recombination frequency, for example, for chromosomes 21 [3].

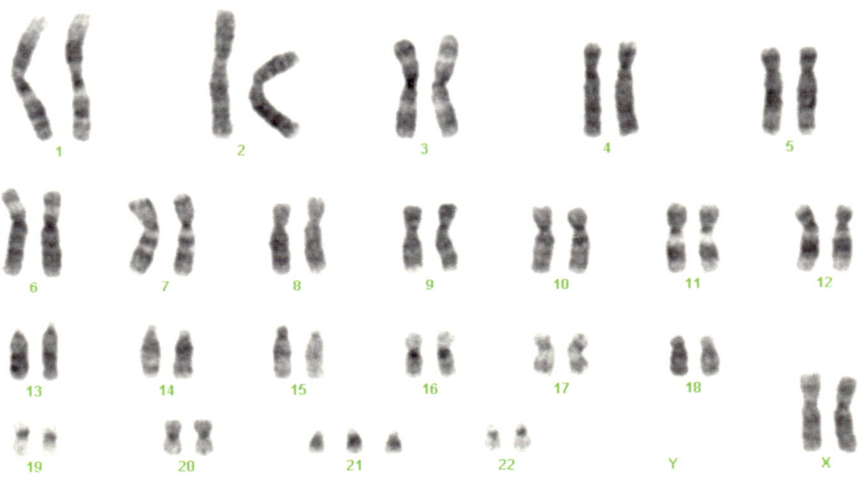

Figure 1. XX,+21 female Down syndrome karyotype demonstrating trisomy 21. (Karyotype prepared by Fatma Soylemez)

Aneuploidy is the second major category of chromosome mutations in which chromosome number is abnormal. An aneuploid is an individual organism whose chromosome number differs from the wild type by part of a chromosome set. Double aneuploidy that leads to trisomy of the two different chromosomes occurs due to accidentally meiotic nondisjunction events; both could have a same or different parental origin. The first case of double aneuploidy (48,XXY,+21) was reported in 1959 by Ford et al [4]. Other double aneuploidy that are found frequently are 48,XXX,+21, 48,XXY,+18 and 48,XXX,+18.

In this chapter, we will discuss double aneuploidies in Down syndrome in the light of the published reports. We will also examine possible underlying mechanism involved in the double aneuploidy.

http://dx.doi.org/10.5772/60438

Syndrome	Karyotype	Main clinical features
Down	Trisomy 21	Short, broad hands with single palmar crease, decreased muscle tone, mental retardation, broad head with characteristic features, open mouth with large tongue, up-slanting eyes
Edwards	Trisomy 18	Multiple congenital malformations of many organs, low-set malformed ears, receding mandible, small eyes, mouth and nose with general elfin appearance, severe mental deficiency, congenital heart defects, horseshoe or double kidney, short sternum, posterior heel prominence
Patau	Trisomy 13	Severe mental deficiency, small eyes, cleft lip and/or palate, extra fingers and toes, cardiac anomalies, midline brain anomalies, genitourinary abnormalities
Turner	45,X	Female with retarded sexual development, usually sterile, short stature, webbing of skin in neck region, cardiovascular abnormalities, hearing impairment, normal intelligence
Klinefelter	47,XXY	Male, infertile with small testes, may have some breast development, tall, mild mental deficiency, long limbs, at risk for educational problems
Triple X	47,XXX	Female with normal genitalia and fertility, at risk for educational and emotional problems, early menopause

Table 1. Clinical features of patients with common autosomal or sex chromosome aneuploidy.

2. Common double aneuploidies involving chromosome 21 and autosomal chromosomes

The simultaneous occurrence of two independent chromosomal anomalies in a given individual has been reported for various combinations of aberrations. Such associations most frequently involve aneuploidy of a sex chromosome and trisomy of an autosome, while double autosomal trisomies are less frequent. The reported cases involving autosome and/or sex chromosome aneuploidy, such as double autosomal trisomy are extremely rare in live newborns.

The data of fourteen previously reported cases with double autosomal trisomy, twelve of them mosaics, may be summarized as follows: The distribution of the maternal ages at birth of the patients was striking: six mothers were younger than 21 years, seven mothers were older than 34 years. In those patients with prevalence of one of the two extra chromosomes in their karyotypes, the corresponding trisomy syndrome also predominated clinically. In those cases with an equal proportion of both additional chromosomes there were as many patients with clinical predominance of the one as of the other trisomy syndrome. Survival beyond the second half of the first year of life was seen only in those patients who showed the clinical picture of mongolism.

2.1. Down and trisomy 18 (Edwards) syndrome

The trisomy 18 syndrome, also known as Edwards syndrome, is a common chromosomal disorder due to the presence of an extra chromosome 18, either full, mosaic trisomy, or partial trisomy 18q. The condition is the second most common autosomal trisomy syndrome after trisomy 21 [5].

The syndrome pattern comprises a recognizable pattern of major and minor anomalies, an increased risk of neonatal and infant mortality, and significant psychomotor and cognitive disability. The main clinical features represent the clues for the diagnosis in the perinatal period and include prenatal growth deficiency, characteristic craniofacial features, distinctive hand posture, nail hypoplasia, short hallux, short sternum, and major malformations (Table 1).

Most authorities have suggested that the extra chromosome is present because of nondisjunction. In parent of origin analyses the extra chromosome is most often of maternal origin, the result of an error during the segregation of chromosomes in meiosis or post zygotic mitosis. About 50% of the nondisjunction errors in oogenesis occur in meiosis II, unlike other human trisomies where the malsegregation is more frequent in meiosis I. In the minority of cases in which the extra chromosome has a paternal origin, the error is the result of a post zygotic error. The cause of nondisjunction is unknown.

Most reported cases of double aneuploidy of Edwards syndrome are Edwards-Turner, Edwards-XXX, Edwards-Klinefelter and Edwards-XYY. However, double aneuploidy involving Down and Edwards syndromes is very rare occurrence because most of them probably are miscarriages (Table 2). Interestingly, the existence of double autosomal trisomy was reported in a newborn child: Down syndrome-trisomy 18 and Down syndrome and trisomy 13 [6].

Karyotype	Phenotype	Reference
48,XX,+18,+21	Edwards/Down Syndrome	Hsu et al, 1965 [7]
48,XX,+18,+21	Edwards/Down Syndrome	Grosse et al, 1977 [8]
48,XX,+18,+21	Edwards/Down Syndrome	Castel et al, 1983 [6]
48,XX,+18,+21	Edwards/Down Syndrome	Reddy et al, 1997 [9]

Table 2. Some examples of double aneuploidy in patients affected with Down and Edwards Syndrome.

2.2. Down and trisomy 13 (Patau) syndrome

Trisomy 13, also called Patau syndrome, is the least common of the major autosomal trisomies with an estimated incidence of 1 in 20 000 live births. Trisomy 13 is associated with advanced maternal age. The extra 13 usually results from a maternal meiotic nondisjunctional error.

http://dx.doi.org/10.5772/60438

Trisomy 13 is a chromosomal condition associated with severe intellectual disability and physical abnormalities in many parts of the body. Individuals with trisomy 13 often have heart defects, brain or spinal cord abnormalities, very small or poorly developed eyes (microphthalmia), extra fingers or toes, an opening in the lip (a cleft lip) with or without an opening in the roof of the mouth (a cleft palate), and weak muscle tone (hypotonia) (Table 1). Owing to severe clinical abnormalities including central nervous system malformations, heart defects, growth retardation and numerous other congenital anomalies. trisomy 13 patients rarely survive the newborn period.

Due to the presence of several life-threatening medical problems, many infants with trisomy 13 die within their first days or weeks of life. Only five percent to 10 percent of children with this condition live past their first year. Like Edwards syndrome many affected pregnancies do not survive to delivery and therefore the incidence in mid pregnancy is higher. Double aneuploidy involving Down and Patau syndromes is very rare occurrence because most of them probably are miscarriages as well as Edwards syndrome (Table 3).

Karyotype	Phenotype	Reference
48,XX,+13,+21	Patau/Down Syndrome	Castel et al, 1983 [6]
48,XX,+13,+21/47,XX,+21	Patau/Down Syndrome mosaic Down Syndrome	Barnett et al, 1987 [10]
48,XX,+13,+21	Patau/Down Syndrome	Reddy et al, 1997 [9]
48,XY,+13,+21	Patau/Down Syndrome	Jenderny, 2014 [11]

Table 3. Some examples of double aneuploidy in patients affected with Down and Patau Syndrome.

3. Common double aneuploidies involving chromosome 21 and sex chromosomes

Sex chromosome abnormalities have less severe clinical anomalies than those associated with comparable autosomal imbalances. This difference can be attributed to genetic inactivation of all but one X-chromosome in those cases where multiple copies are present, and the relatively low gene content of the Y-chromosome. Sex chromosome aneuploidy is relatively common, with overall frequency of about 1 in 500 live births. Some (XXX, XXY, XYY) are relatively frequent in newborns but rare in spontaneous abortions. Monosomy X (Turner syndrome), in contrast, is one of the most common chromosome abnormalities seen in spontaneous abortions but relatively rare in newborns.

3.1. Down and Turner syndrome (45,X)

Turner syndrome, a disorder in females characterized by the absence of all or part of a normal second sex chromosome, leads to a constellation of physical findings that often includes congenital lymphedema, short stature, and gonadal dysgenesis (Table 1). Turner's syndrome occurs in 1 in 2500 to 1 in 3000 live-born girls. Approximately half have monosomy X (45,X), and 5 to 10 percent have a duplication (isochromosome) of the long arm of one X (46,X,i(Xq)). Most of the rest have mosaicism for 45,X, with one or more additional cell lineages.

The clinical features range from a severe phenotypic character with short stature, gonadal dysgenesis and different malformations to an isolated mild reduction in final height or premature ovarian failure. The most visible phenotype is the short stature, which has been reported in up to 98 % of all Turner syndrome patients. Peripheral lymphedema dorsally of the hands and feet may be the initial presenting sign of Turner syndrome and is found in approximately one-third of affected infants. Turner's syndrome should be suspected in any newborn girl with edema or hypoplastic left heart or coarctation of the aorta, since the frequency of both conditions is increased among children with Turner's syndrome. In the last decade, the association between aortic dissection and Turner syndrome has been increasingly recognized with several reports of sudden death. In most other patients with Turner's syndrome, the condition is diagnosed either in adolescence when they fail to enter puberty or in adulthood because of recurrent pregnancy loss.

Most of Turner syndrome cases have mosaicism with Down syndrome. However, double aneuploidy involving Down and Turner syndromes is a rare occurrence (Table 4). The patients reported to have combined Down and Turner syndromes, fundamentally usually different forms of chromosome mosaicism have been noted and all have been mosaic with respect to monosomy X. Townes et al reported the first example of a Turner-Down patient in whom there was no X mosaicism [12].

Karyotype	Phenotype	Reference
46,X,+21	Turner/Down Syndrome	Townes et al, 1975 [12]
46,X,+21/47,XX,+21	Turner/Down Syndrome mosaic Down Syndrome	MacFaul, 1981 [14]
46,X,+21	Turner/Down Syndrome	Ruangdaraganon, 1993 [16]
46,X,+21	Turner/Down Syndrome	Jaruratanasirikul et al, 1995 [13]
46,X,+21/47,XX,+21	Turner/Down Syndrome mosaic Down Syndrome	Zaki et al, 2005 [15]
46,X,+21	Turner/Down Syndrome	Jenderny, 2014 [11]

Table 4. Some examples of double aneuploidy in patients affected with Down and Turner Syndrome

One of the first reports with double aneuploidy (Turner-Down) was reported that the first example of a Turner-Down patient in whom there is no X mosaicism [12]. The case of an 8 month-old female infant with non-mosaic Down-Turner double aneuploidy was reported by Jaruratanasirikul et al [13]. She had Down faces without stigmata of Turner syndrome.

Down's/Turner's mosaic is a rare chromosomal abnormality, occurring in about 1 in 2 000 000 births. Two babies with Down's/Turner's mosaic karyotype was reported that 2 babies born with this disorder in each of whom chromosomal analysis of amniotic fluid had mistakenly identified the fetus as a normal male [14]. The infant had the facial appearance of a Down

http://dx.doi.org/10.5772/60438

syndrome. She was markedly hypotonic with a low hairline, and had pronounced webbing of the neck. The heart was normal. Karyotype was 46,X+21/47XX+21. The 46,X+21 was present in 12% of the cultured cells. At age 11 months she had the appearance typical of Down syndrome together with some webbing of the neck. Mother was 35 years old. Same investigators reported another patient who had a baby with Down/Turner aneuploidy. Mother was 38 years old. The amniotic fluid karyotype was thought to be 46,XY. A girl weighing 1750 g was delivered at 36 weeks' gestation by caesarean section performed for intrauterine growth retardation. The infant had the facial appearance of Down's syndrome, a large clitoris, puffy hands and feet, and for a few days was cyanosed in air, and had a cardiac murmur. There was a single palmar crease and talipes on the right. She died from bronchopneumonia aged 15 weeks. The karyotype obtained in the neonatal period was 47,XX+21/46,X+21. Zaki and colleagues recently represented a female, mosaic (46,X,+21/47,XX,+21) where monosomy X was detected only by FISH in 15 percentages of cells, nevertheless, stigmata of Turner syndrome was more obvious in this patient [15].

3.2. Down and Klinefelter syndrome (47,XXY)

Klinefelter syndrome is a chromosomal condition that affects male physical and cognitive development. Its signs and symptoms vary among affected individuals. The incidence of 48,XXY,+21 in the general population is 0.4 to 0.9 per 10,000 male births. Unlike Turner syndrome, males with Klinefelter syndrome are not usually detected in the newborn period. These individuals are generally normal in appearance before puberty. After puberty they are frequently ascertained in infertility clinics or identified by their small testes, breast enlargement and tall stature. Affected individuals typically have small testes that do not produce as much testosterone as usual. Some affected individuals also have genital differences including undescended testes, the opening of the urethra on the underside of the penis (hypospadias), or an unusually micropenis (Table 1). Significant mental retardation is not part of this syndrome but patients have a higher incidence of educational and emotional problems.

Klinefelter and his colleagues (1942) described a characteristic syndrome in nine male patients who had gynecomastia and a specific form of hypogonadism comprising small testes with hyalinized seminiferous tubules and absent spermatogenesis but with intact Leyding cells. This syndrome is now well established in clinical practice and contributes significantly to infertility in the male.

Most Klinefelter patients have a 47,XXY karyotype (Figure 2). At least 10% have mosaicism involving normal 46,XY cells plus another population of cells with two or more X chromosomes. Mosaic patients have more variable clinical features and occasionally may have relatively normal testicular development. Cytogenetic and molecular data have indicated that 47,XXY is equally likely to result from a maternal or paternal meiotic nondisjunctional error. Maternally derived cases are associated with maternal age. Variants of Klinefelter syndrome include those patients with more than two X-chromosomes, multiple X-chromosome mosaicism and multiple Y-chromosomes. The presence of additional X-chromosomes is associated with increasing severity of clinical abnormalities including mental retardation, sexual development and skeletal anomalies.

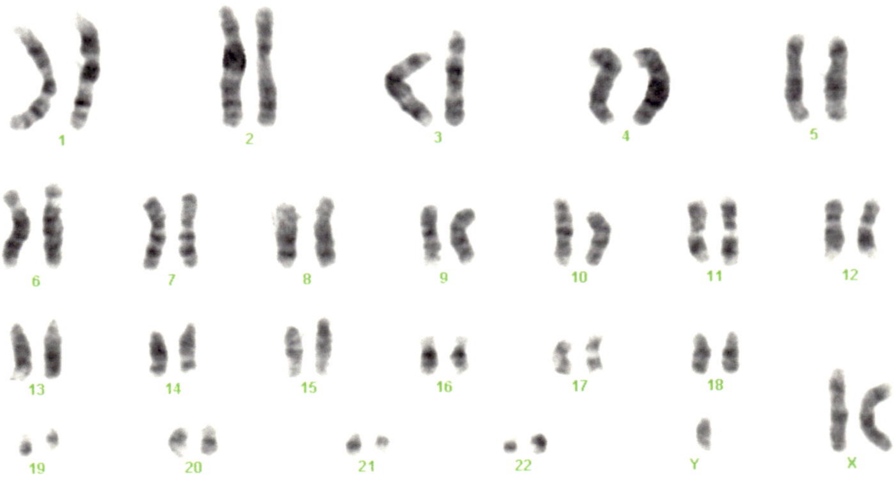

Figure 2. XXY Klinefelter syndrome karyotype (Karyotype prepared by Fatma Soylemez).

Trisomy 21 and numerical sex chromosome anomalies are common chromosome disorders. Down syndrome is the most common chromosomal abnormality in humans with an incidence of one in 770 live births. Although it is the most intensively studied human chromosomal abnormality, little is known about its cause and only advanced maternal age is confirmed as a risk factor [17]. On the other hand, Klinefelter syndrome is the most common disorder of sex chromosomes in humans, with prevalence of one in 500 males. The classic form is the most common chromosomal disorder, in which there is one extra X chromosome resulting in the karyotype of 47,XXY [18]. Double aneuploidy was first described in a patient with both Down and Klinefelter (48, XXY,+21) syndromes. This is also the most commonly described double aneuploidy. The karyotype is shown on Figure 3 [19].

The coincidence rate of both Down and Klinefelter syndromes in the same individual is estimated to lie in the range 0.27 to 0.7 × 10-5 [20]. On the other hand, lower values of XXY pattern recorded in older boys and men with Down syndrome suggest that there might be an increased selection against these individuals after birth [21]. Several cases of double aneuploidy of XXY and trisomy 21 have been published since the first report by Ford et al. (Table 5).

Pediatric cardiologists are familiar with screening of babies with Down syndrome for congenital heart defects, expecting in approximately 50% to find a heart defect, typically atrioventricular septal defect. However, in children diagnosed with Klinefelter syndrome, a chronic heart disease has only rarely been reported. Shen et al reported one case of 48,XXY,+21 karyotype with chronic heart disease. The phenotypic characteristics of the 4-month-old child had showed the presence of features typical of mongoloid slant. Also, Doppler echocardiogram detection has been showed atrial septal and ventricular septal defects with patent ductus arteriosus, pulmonary hypertension and mild tricuspid regurgitation [22]. Similarly, a 14-month-old boy was reported with double aneuploidy and a double aortic arch suffered from frequently recurrent severe feeding and respiratory problems [23].

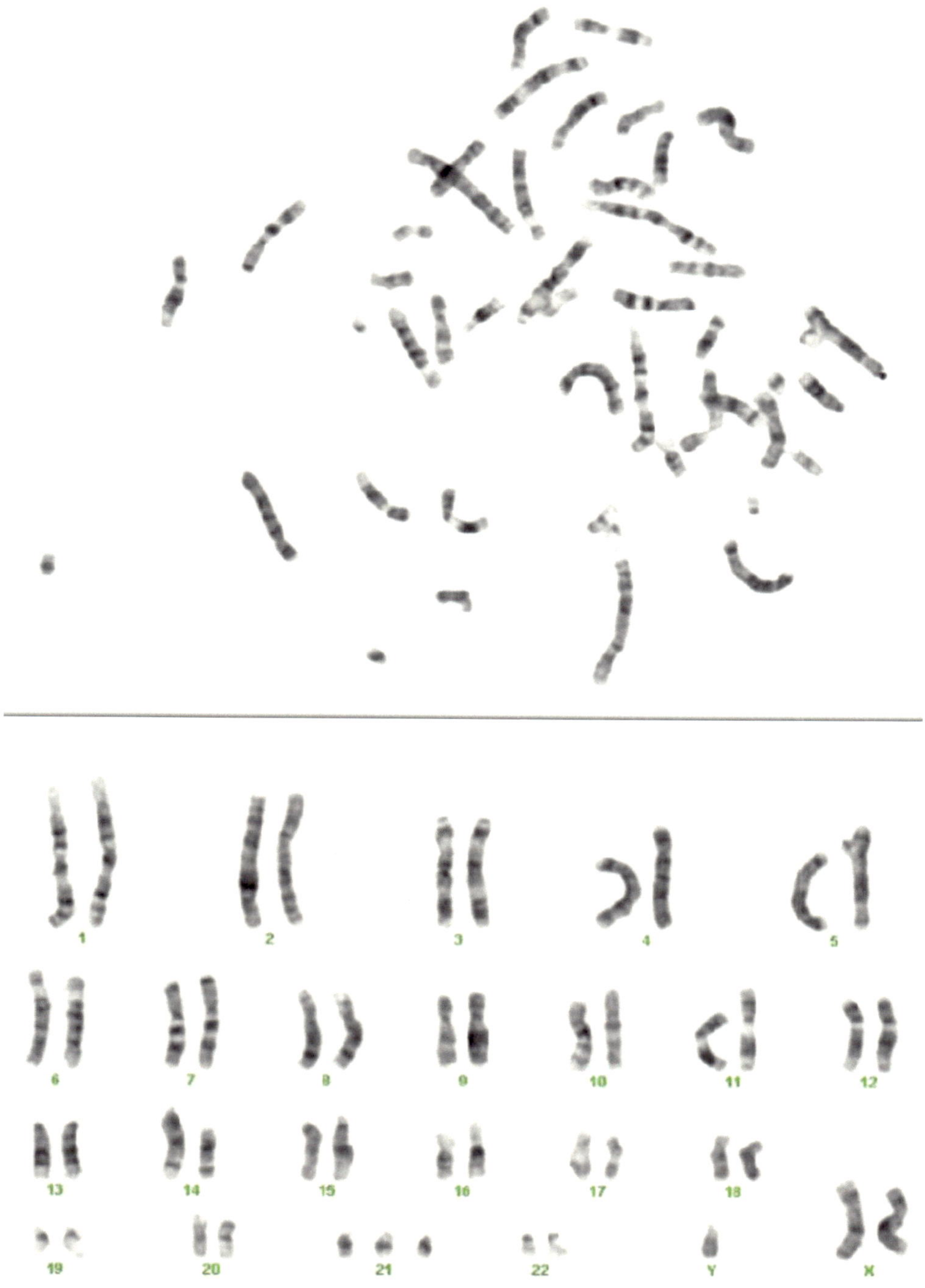

Figure 3. GTG-banded karyotype of the case showing double aneuploidy - 48,XXY,+21. (Karyotype prepared by Fatma Soylemez.)

Karyotype	Phenotype	Reference
48,XXY,+21	Klinefelter/Down Syndrome	Ford et al, 1959 [4]
48,XXY,+21	Klinefelter/Down Syndrome	Harnden et al, 1960 [33]
48,XXY,+21	Klinefelter/Down Syndrome	Lanman et al, 1960 [34]
48,XXY,+21	Klinefelter/Down Syndrome	Hustinx et al, 1961 [35]
48,XXY,+21	Klinefelter/Down Syndrome	Gelderen and Hustinx, 1961 [36]
48,XXY,+21	Klinefelter/Down Syndrome	Hamerton et al, 1961 [26]
48,XXY,+21	Klinefelter/Down Syndrome	Milcou and Mainanesco, 1963 [37]
48,XXY,+21	Klinefelter/Down Syndrome	Court Brown et al, 1964 [38]
48,XXY,+21	Klinefelter/Down Syndrome	Pfeiffer, 1964 [39]
48,XXY,+21	Klinefelter/Down Syndrome	Taylor and Moores, 1967 [27]
47,XXY/48,XXY,+21	Klinefelter/Down Syndrome-Mosaic	Yamaguchi et al, 1989 [20]
48,XXY,+21	Klinefelter/Down Syndrome	Al Awadi et al, 1998 [25]
48,XXY,+21	Klinefelter/Down Syndrome	Iliopoulus et al, 2004 [24]
48,XXY,+21	Klinefelter/Down Syndrome	Cyril et al, 2005 [40]
48,XXY,+21	Klinefelter/Down Syndrome	Glass et al, 2006 [17]
48,XXY,+21	Klinefelter/Down Syndrome	Akbas, Soylemez et al, 2008 [19]
48,XXY,+21	Klinefelter/Down Syndrome	Karaman and Kabalar, 2008 [41]
48,XXY,+21	Klinefelter/Down Syndrome	Biselli et al, 2009 [42]
48,XXY,+21	Klinefelter/Down Syndrome	Jeanty and Turner, 2009 [43]
48,XXY,+21	Klinefelter/Down Syndrome	Gerretsen et al, 2009 [23]
48,XXY,+21	Klinefelter/Down Syndrome	Shen et al, 2012 [22]
48,XXY,+21	Klinefelter/Down Syndrome	Shu et al, 2013 [24]
48,XXY,+21	Klinefelter/Down Syndrome	Mishra et al, 2014 [44]

Table 5. Some examples of double aneuploidy in patients affected with Down and Klinefelter Syndrome.

Shu et al recently presented a neonate with a double aneuploidy associated with congenital heart defect suffered from cyanosis after birth. The patient had typical features of Down syndrome including hypertelorism, slightly lowest ears with protruding pinna (Figure 4). Doppler echocardiography has been indicated complex congenital heart disease with an ostium secundum atrial septal defect, enlarged right ventricle, and mild tricuspid valve regurgitation. Until now, only eight cases of double aneuploidy associated with CHD defect has been reported [24].

http://dx.doi.org/10.5772/60438

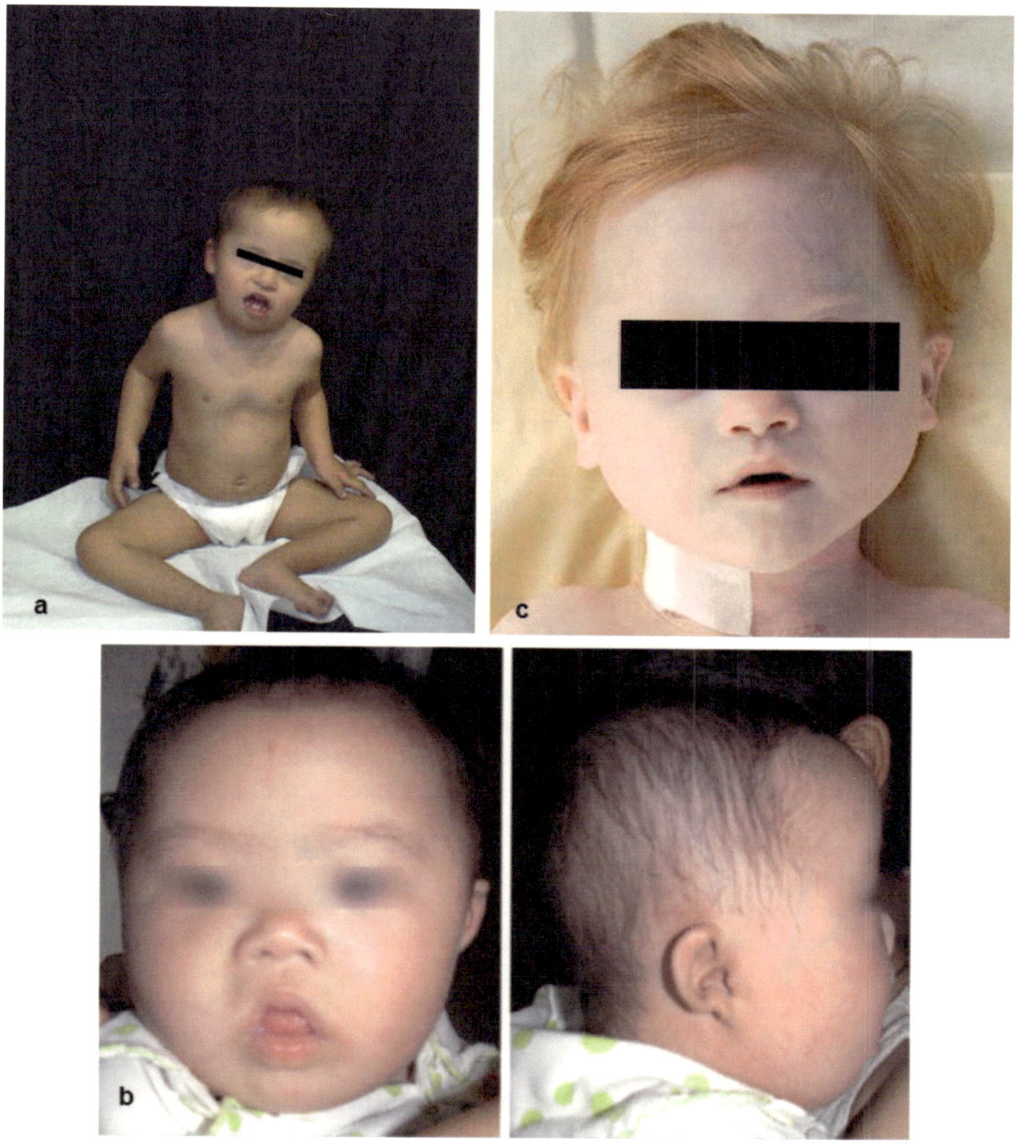

Figure 4. Facial dysmorphic features of the children with karyotype 48,XXY,+21, reveals signs of Down syndrome. a) [19], b) [22], c) [23]

This abnormality has also been described in a pair of monozygotic twins [25]. Further, both the sibs of the proband showing 48,XXY,+21 were found to exhibit trisomy 21 in yet another study [26]. Hamerton et al have summarized the data on the frequency of 48,XXY,+21 males and concluded that the expected incidence of double trisomics based on chance association should be about 0.31×10^{-5} live-born males [27]. In six sex chromatin surveys of the newborn 23.229 live-born males were studied; 47 of these were chromatin positive and two were double trisomics (48,XXY,+21), an incidence of $8.62x10^{-5}$ [28]. This was 18 times higher than the indirect estimate for the general population and 30 times higher than the expected frequency based on chance association. These figures suggested that there was a much higher incidence of double trisomics at birth than would be expected by chance; the most satisfactory explanation for the reduced incidence among older groups was that double trisomics had a much higher mortality during the early years of life than the primary trisomics.

The association of Klinefelter Syndrome and Down syndrome in the same siblings has already been referred to and would be expected by chance although this is more difficult to establish. In particular, three of them, trisomy 21, trisomy 18 and trisomy 13 are the most frequently seen autosomal aneuploidies. Other commonly seen gonosomal aneuploidies are Turner syndrome, Klinefelter syndrome and its variants, poly X syndromes and poly Y syndromes. However, neonatal survey data has revealed that the incidence of XXY and trisomy 21 double trisomy at birth is higher than expected from the incidence of either alone [28].

The prenatal mortality rate of Downs-Klinefelter syndrome has not been extensively studied. Mutton et al found that 35% (6 of 17) of double aneuploidy cases that included an additional chromosome 21 died in utero [29]. Kovaleva and Mutton reported 2 miscarriages in 10 cases of prenatally diagnosed 48,XXY,+21, giving a mortality rate of 20%. Compared with either condition alone, the survival rate for the combination of XXY and trisomy 21 appears to be intermediary [30]. Forrester and Merz reported 1 death in utero (3.5%) in 28 cases of Klinefelter syndrome [31]. Bojesen et al reported no intrauterine deaths in 49 fetuses with prenatally diagnosed Klinefelter syndrome [32]. These data excluded terminations of pregnancies. Since the first reported cases of double aneuploidy with 48, XXY,+21 karyotype [20, 28, 33-40], many cases with Down and Klinefelter syndrome in the same individual has been reported in the literature, some of them very new [17,19, 22-26,41-44] (Table 5).

3.3. Down and Triple X syndrome (47,XXX)

Triple X syndrome, also called trisomy X or 47,XXX, is characterized by the presence of an additional X chromosome in each of a female's cells. The frequency of 47,XXX in newborn females is about 1 in 1000 and is associated with maternal age. Most XXX females are clinically normal with normal gonadal function and fertility. Although females with this condition may be taller than average, this chromosomal change typically causes no unusual physical features. Most females with triple X syndrome have normal sexual development and are able to conceive children. However, there is an increased risk for learning disabilities, reduction in performance IQ, menstrual problems and early menopause (Table 1). Triple X syndrome is associated with an increased risk of learning disabilities and delayed development of speech and language skills. Delayed development of motor skills such as sitting and walking, weak muscle tone (hypotonia), and behavioral and emotional difficulties are also possible, but these characteristics vary widely among affected girls and women (Figure 5). Seizures or kidney abnormalities occur in about 10 percent of affected females. Thus, the clinical manifestations are of trisomy 21 alone in many cases reported that Triple X syndrome/Down syndrome double aneuploidy. Trisomy-21 and triple-X in the same individual has been reported earlier [45, 46] and more recently [47-52] and phenotypic features of classical Down syndrome were only seen. However, strabismus, periorbital swelling, scanty eyebrows and microganthia have not been observed in these reports (Table 6).

http://dx.doi.org/10.5772/60438

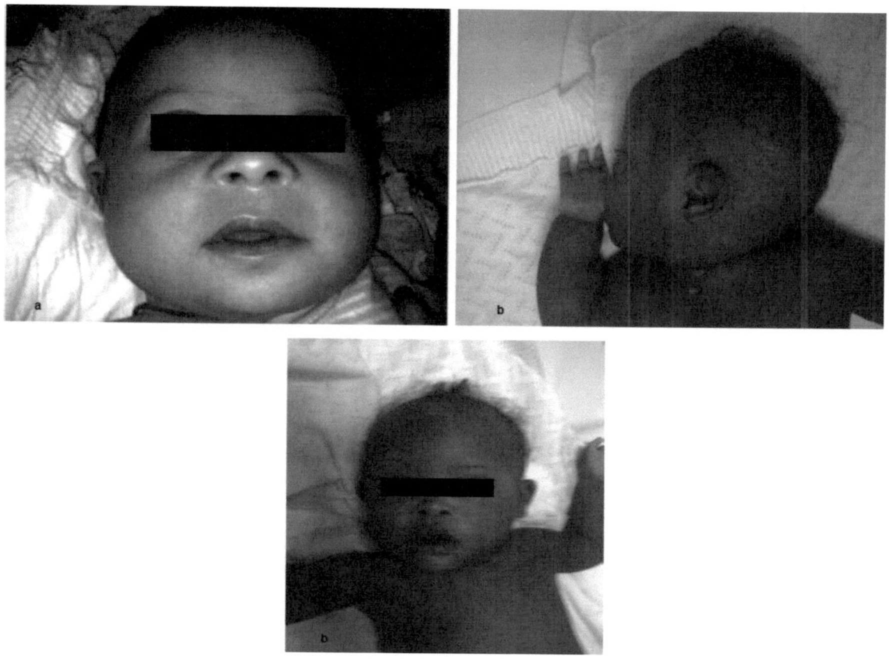

Figure 5. Phenotype of the child with karyotype 48,XXX,+21 showing characteristic faces with low set ears and short neck. a) [51], b) [52]

Sheth et al reported a case of double aneuploidy showing trisomy 21 and triple-X chromosome in a case of Down syndrome born to young non-consanguineous parents. The child presented with strabismus, periorbital swelling, scanty eyebrows and microganthia in addition to Down features. Molecular characterization had shown the maternal origin of double aneuploidy with trisomy 21 at meiosis-II and triple-X at meiosis-I [51].

Karyotype	Phenotype	Reference
48,XXX,+21	Double chromatin positive female with Down Syndrome	Day et al, 1963 [45]
48,XXX,+21	Double chromatin positive female with Down Syndrome	Yunis et al, 1964 [46]
48,XXX,+21	Triple X/Down Syndrome	Park et al, 1995 [47]
48,XXX,+21	Triple X/Down Syndrome	Devlin and Morrison, 2004 [48]
48,XXX,+21	Triple X/Down Syndrome	Balwan et al, 2008 [49]
48,XXX,+21	Triple X/Down Syndrome	Guzel et al, 2009 [50]
48,XXX,+21	Triple X/Down Syndrome	Sheth et al, 2011 [51]
48,XXX,+21	Triple X/Down Syndrome	Uwineza et al, 2012 [52]

Table 6. Some examples of double aneuploidy in patients affected with Down and Triple X Syndrome

3.4. Down and 47,XYY syndrome

47,XYY syndrome is characterized by an extra copy of the Y chromosome in each of a male's cells. Approximately 1 in 1000 newborn males have a 47,XYY karyotype. Although most 47,XYY patients are clinically normal, they tend to be taller than normal and have an increased tendency for behavioral and learning problems as children and young adults. Y-chromosome aneuploidy results from paternal meiotic nondisjunction and is not associated with maternal age. Although males with this condition may be taller than average, this chromosomal change typically causes no unusual physical features. Most males with 47,XYY syndrome have normal sexual development and are able to father children. 47,XYY syndrome is associated with an increased risk of learning disabilities and delayed development of speech and language skills. Delayed development of motor skills such as sitting and walking, weak muscle tone (hypotonia), hand tremors or other involuntary movements (motor tics), and behavioral and emotional difficulties are also possible (Table 1). These characteristics vary widely among affected boys and men. A small percentage of males with 47,XYY syndrome are diagnosed with autistic spectrum disorders, which are developmental conditions that affect communication and social interaction.

Most cases of 47,XYY syndrome are not inherited. The chromosomal change usually occurs as a random event during the formation of sperm cells. An error in cell division called nondisjunction can result in sperm cells with an extra copy of the Y chromosome. If one of these atypical reproductive cells contributes to the genetic makeup of a child, the child will have an extra Y chromosome in each of the body's cells. The XYY occurs when 24YY spermatozoa are formed due to nondisjunction either at paternal meiosis II or mitosis. Unlike Down syndrome, the XYY is not associated with increased parental age. The only consistent phenotypic feature associated with the XYY syndrome is tall stature, which becomes evident at about 5-6 years of age. These children may have learning difficulties, attention deficits, hyperactivity and increased aggressiveness. However, the behavioral changes appear to be variable and may be modified by the environment in which these children live. Therefore, it is important to recognize the XYY abnormality at the earliest so that these children can be evaluated periodically and given appropriate care and interventions for learning and behavioral needs.

Karyotype	Phenotype	Reference
48,XYY,+21	47,XYY/Down Syndrome	Verresen et al, 1965 [53]
48,XYY,+21	47,XYY/Down Syndrome	Migeon, 1965 [54]
48,XYY,+21	47,XYY/Down Syndrome	Uchida et al, 1966 [55]
47,XYY,+21	47,XYY/Down Syndrome	Al-Aish MS et al, 1971 [56]
47,XYY,+21/47,XY,+21	47,XYY /Down Syndrome mosaic Down Syndrome	Schwanitz et al, 1978 [57]
47,XYY,+21	47,XYY/Down Syndrome	Reddy, 1997 [58]
47,XYY,+21	47,XYY/Down Syndrome	Parmar et al, 2002 [59]
47,XYY,+21	47,XYY /Down Syndrome	Koken et al, 2011 [60]
47,XYY,+21/47,XY,+21	47,XYY/Down Syndrome mosaic Down Syndrome	Parihar et al, 2013 [61]

Table 7. Some examples of double aneuploidy in patients affected with Down and 47,XYY Syndrome

http://dx.doi.org/10.5772/60438

Although etiological predisposing factor for 48,XYY,+21 is not known, there are reported several cases of karyotype with 48,XYY,+21 since 1970's [53-57] (Table 7). Fewer than 40 cases of Down syndrome with XYY have been reported until date, only one of which has mosaicism for XYY. Reddy observed only 22 cases of double aneuploidy, such as XXY and 21 trisomy among 3024 spontaneous abortuses that the frequency even less than expected if the two aneuploidy events were independent of each other. They also occurred at an older mean maternal age [58]. Koken et al presented the patient had typical features of Down syndrome, however, phenotypic features of XYY was not present (Figure 6). In addition, the patient also had atrial septal defect, multiple trabecular small ventricular septal defect, and moderate degree of pulmonary hypertension [60]. Parihar et al reported a 5-year-old boy with the clinical features of Down syndrome. Cytogenetic analysis has been showed a mosaicism for a double aneuploidy, Down syndrome and XYY. The karyotype was 47, XY,+21(19)/48, XYY,+21(6),ish XYY (DXZ1 × 1, DYZ1 × 2) [61].

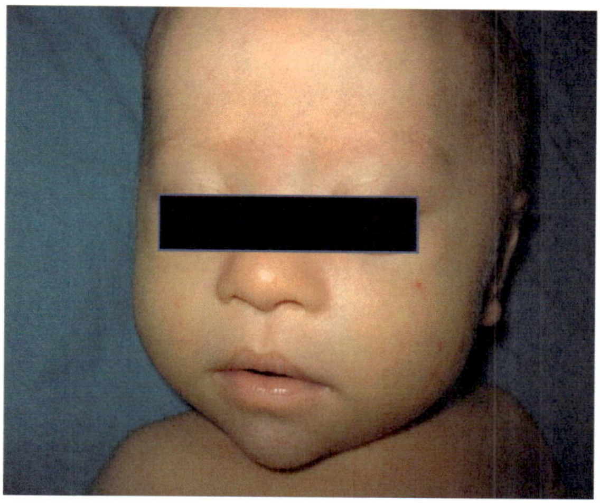

Figure 6. Phenotype of the child with karyotype 48,XYY,+21, reveals signs of Down syndrome [60-Koken et al, 2011].

4. Results

It has been over 50 years since trisomy 21 was identified as the cause of Down's syndrome, providing the first link between a clinical disorder and a chromosome abnormality. In the intervening half-century, the importance of numerical chromosome abnormalities to human disease pathology has been well-documented. Taken together, these studies established aneuploidy as the leading known cause of congenital birth defects and miscarriage and demonstrated that most aneuploid conceptuses perish in utero.

The occurrence of double aneuploidy i.e. the existence of two chromosomal abnormalities in the same individual is an uncommon phenomenon. Although aneuploidies are common structural chromosomal abnormalities, double aneuploidies involving chromosomes 21 and sex and autosomal chromosomes are very rare. Trisomy 21 and numerical sex chromosome anomalies are common chromosomal disorders, with a birth incidence of 1:700 to 1:2,500 respectively [30]. The chances of two chromosomal anomalies occurring in a single conceptus are a rare event and the reported incidence varies from 0.21% to 2.8% in spontaneous miscarriages subjected to cytogenetic study [50]. In 1959, the first case with autosomal and sex chromosomal anomalies, 48,XXY,+21, was presented by Ford et al [4].

Various double aneuploidy associations are summarized in Tables above. The most frequently reported type of double aneuploidy is the 48,XXY,+21; other types include 48,XYY,+21. In general, the double aneuploidies which involve the sex chromosomes as well as 21-trisomy have phenotypic features representative of both aneuploidy conditions. These usually have the features of both conditions although the more serious condition usually masks the less serious. The presence of an associated sex chromosome abnormality in children with Down syndrome may not be clinically evident until puberty.

The existence of two chromosomal abnormalities in the same individual is relatively a rare phenomenon. Double aneuploidy leading to trisomy and/or monosomy of two different chromosomes arises because of two meiotic nondisjunctional events. Both these aneuploidies could have the same or different parental origin [62]. Double aneuploidy leading to trisomy and / or monosomy of two different chromosomes arises because of two meiotic nondisjunctional events. Both aneuploidies arise as a result of nondisjunction in maternal meiosis II [47] and these results support the hypothesis that a segregation defect at the cellular level may cause nondisjunction involving more than one chromosome. Most reported cases of double aneuploidy are presented in the form of spontaneous abortions. The reported cases involving autosome and/or sex chromosome aneuploidy, such as double autosomal trisomy and autosomal trisomy with sex chromosome monosomy or trisomy, are extremely rare in live newborns. These syndromes include Edwards-Down, Down-Klinefelter, Down-Turner mosaicism, Down-XYY, Patau-Klinefelter, Edwards-Turner mosaicism, Edwards-XXX, Edwards-Klinefelter, and Edwards-XYY. A rare case of double chromosome aneuploidy including Edwards syndrome (trisomy 18) and Klinefelter syndrome was described highlighting the patient's longer life span. Most cases of double aneuploidies in live births involve the sex chromosomes combined with either trisomy 13, 18 or 21, i.e. XXX/18, XXX/21, XXY/13, XXY/18, XXY/21, XYY/13, XYY/18 and XYY/21.

Double aneuploidies are observed in 0.21-2.8% of the aborted fetuses [63]. For women 35 years and older, the rate of trisomy 21 is increased to 1 per 120 pregnancies when data from 2 sources are combined. The rate of Klinefelter syndrome in pregnancies carried by women 35 years or older is 1 per 787.41 By multiplying the individual frequencies, the expected frequency of 48,XXY,+21 would be 1 per 94,440 pregnancies. Caron et al found 1 case of 48,XXY,+21 in 24,901 amniocentesis performed for advanced maternal age (≥35 years), which is a 3.8-fold increase over the expected rate [64]. The nonrandom aspect of double aneuploidy provides evidence that a hereditary predisposition to nondisjunction exists, with one chromosomal imbalance increasing the risk of another to occur, which suggests that both events arise from the same parent. Nondisjunction in cases of double trisomy has been found to be entirely maternal in origin, entirely paternal in origin, and both maternal and paternal in origin. In such cases in which the additional chromosomes originate from different parents, the two errors may be coincidental and unrelated to a genetically determined nondisjunction. Abnormal separation of chromosomes may occur in older individuals because of dysfunction of structures related to chromosome separation, such as the spindle apparatus and kinetochore. Among 28 reports of 48,XXY,+21, which include 36 cases with known parental ages, Kovaleva and Mutton found that the risk for 48,XXY,+21 was age dependent, with a mean maternal age of 33 years and a mean paternal age of 38 years [30].

Trisomy 21, resulting in Down Syndrome (DS), is the most common autosomal trisomy among live-born infants and is caused mainly by nondisjunction of chromosome 21 within oocytes. Risk factors for nondisjunction depend on the parental origin and type of meiotic error. For errors in the oocyte, increased maternal age and altered patterns of recombination are highly associated with nondisjunction. Studies of normal meiotic events in humans have shown that recombination clusters in regions referred to as hotspots. In addition, GC content, CpG fraction, Poly(A)/Poly(T) fraction and gene density have been found to be significant predictors of the placement of sex-averaged recombination in the human genome. The results from early studies demonstrated that most aneuploidies are due to errors in maternal meiosis and that increasing maternal age is a powerful contributor to the occurrence of aneuploidy. However, studies during the past 10-15 years have also implicated events that occur at the onset of female meiosis in the fetal ovary and during the protracted dictyate arrest. The duration of the division (10 to 50 years and beyond) provides ample opportunity for errors to occur and to accumulate, which is a feature that has been the basis of a number of hypotheses to explain the maternal age effect. Indeed, the emerging picture indicates that aneuploidy is not due to a single causal factor but involves a complex constellation of effects that begins in utero, continues throughout the reproductive lifespan of the woman, is exacerbated by age and is facilitated by the unique features of cell cycle control in the oocyte.

Trisomics and monosomic (aneuploid) embryos account for at least 10% of human pregnancies and, for women nearing the end of their reproductive lifespan, the incidence may exceed 50%. The errors that lead to aneuploidy almost always occur in the oocyte but, despite intensive investigation, the underlying molecular basis has remained elusive. Increased maternal age and altered number and location of recombination events have been found to be associated with maternal meiotic errors involving chromosome 21 [65]. The overwhelming majority of trisomy 21, or Down syndrome, is caused by the failure of chromosomes to separate properly during meiosis, also known as chromosome nondisjunction. As nondisjunction is the leading cause of pregnancy loss, mental retardation and birth defects, it is imperative that we understand the biology underlying this phenomenon. Characteristics of chromosome 21 nondisjunction are typical of many of the other human autosomes. That is, the overwhelming majority is due to errors during oogenesis: at least 90% of cases have chromosome 21 nondisjunction are due to maternal meiotic errors.

Whereas there was no obvious maternal age association with recombination patterns among normally disjoining chromosomes 21, there was a significant one among maternal MI and "MII" errors. One set of observations provides evidence for specific recombination patterns being the proximal cause of nondisjunction, while the others suggest an interaction between specific recombination patterns and maternal age-related risk factors. Specifically, the absence of recombination or the presence of a single recombinant event near the telomere of 21q are associated with maternal meiosis I (MI) errors and these associations appear to be independent of the age of the oocyte (i.e., maternal age at the time of birth of the infant with trisomy 21). Meiosis II (MII) errors appear to be driven by different age and recombination traits: MII errors are associated with the placement of a recombinant event near the centromere of 21q and this association increases with increasing age of the oocyte.

Nondisjunction could be possibly attributed to genetic, environmental or combined factors. Theoretically genes predisposing to increased nondisjunction can be classified in several different ways: a) Gene(s) producing nondisjunction of a specific chromosome (e.g. chromosome 21), b) Gene(s) that can predispose to nondisjunction of different autosome/sex chromosomes in the same individual, or in sibs, due to, parental and/or post zygotic or post systic nondisjunction "double aneuploidy" (such as, 48,XX, or XY,+21; 48,XXY,+21; 46,X,+21). The occurrence of double aneuploidy would not prove the existence of predisposition gene(s). Such outcome resulting from parental mosaicism has been demonstrated in some families with >2 trisomy 21 sibs. Familial double aneuploidy is very rare. However, the occurrence of aneuploidy for different chromosomes is better evidence for genetic predisposition although environmental factors could also be invoked as a possible cause. Amniocentesis and live birth data provide little evidence for a strong double aneuploidy effect although a weak effect cannot be excluded. Studies in abortions are suggestive of genetic mosaicism in double aneuploidy.

In conclusion, since the first description of a case of double aneuploidy with 48, XXY,+21 karyotype, approximately 385 cases with double aneuploidy are reported in the literature. Autosomal double trisomies are observed in spontaneous abortions but are rarely reported in live born infants. Most double aneuploidies are associated with an increased maternal age, abnormal sonogram, and pregnancy loss at a very early gestational age. However, sex chromosome aneuploidy and trisomies involving chromosomes 16, 18, and 21 can survive for longer gestation. The mechanism underlying the origin of double aneuploidy is unclear. It is hypothesized that double aneuploidy results either from two nondisjunctional events in gametogenesis or a single nondisjunctional event in a trisomics zygote. The published literature shows that there is no specific chromosome association in double aneuploidy formation; however, the most frequently involved chromosomes are the sex chromosomes and acrocentric chromosomes.

Author details

Fatma Soylemez

Address all correspondence to: soylemez_fatma@yahoo.com

University of Avrasya, Department of Molecular Biology and Genetics, Trabzon, Turkey

References

[1] Luthardt F, Keitges E. Chromosomal Syndromes and Genetic Disease. The Quarterly Review of Biology 2001; 79 (1): 69-70.

[2] Sherman SL, Allen EG, Bean LH, Freeman SB. Epidemiology of Down sydrome. Mental Retardation and Developmental Disabilities Research Reviews 2007; 13: 221-227.

[3] Sherman SL, Petersen MB, Freeman SB. Nondisjunction of chromosome 21 in maternal meiosis I: evidence for a maternal age-dependent mechanism involving reduced recombination. Hum Mol Genet 1994; 3: 1529-1535.

[4] Ford CE, Jones KW, Miller OJ, Mittwoch U, Penrose LS, Ridler M et al. The chromosomes in a patient showing both mongolism and the Klinefelter syndrome. Lancet 1959; 1: 709-710.

[5] Carey JC. Trisomy 18 and trisomy 13 syndromes. Management of Genetic Syndromes, Second Edition 2005; 555-568.

[6] Castel Y, Le Marec B, Toudic L, Lemarchand M, Cosson JP. Association of trisomy 21 and gonosomal trisomy. Apropos of 2 cases. Pediatrie. 1983; 38 (4): 235-41.

[7] Hsu LY, Schwanger AJ, Nemhauser I, Sobel EH. A case of double autosomal trisomy with mosaicism: 48/XX (Trisomy 18+21) and 46/XX. J Pediatr. 1965 ;66: 1055-60.

[8] Grosse KP, Schwanitz G. Double autosomal trisomy: case report (48, XX, +18, +21) and review of the literature. J Ment Defic Res 1977; 21: 299-308.

[9] Reddy KS. Double trisomy and spontaneous abortions. Hum Genet 1997; 101: 339-345.

[10] Barnett SH, Jhaveri M, Gertner M. Double autosomal trisomy mosaicism: 47,XY, +21/48,XY,+13,+21. Am J Med Genet. 1987; 28 (2): 501-502.

[11] Jenderny J. Chromosome aberrations in a large series of spontaneous miscarriages in the German population and review of the literature. Mol Cytogenet. 2014; 5 ;7-38.

[12] Townes PL, White MR, Stiffler SJ, Goh K. Double aneuploidy. Turner-Down syndrome. Am J Dis Child. 1975; 129 (9): 1062-5.

[13] Jaruratanasirikul S, Jinorose U. An infant with Down-Turner double aneuploidy: a case report and literature review. J Med Assoc Thai. 1995; 78 (2): 108-12.

[14] MacFaul R, Turner T, Mason MK. Down's/Turner's mosaicism. Double aneuploidy as a rare cause of missed prenatal diagnosis of chromosomal abnormality. Arch Dis Child. 1981; 56 (12): 962-963.

[15] Zaki MS, Kamel AA, El-Ruby M. Double aneuploidy in three Egyptian patients: Down-Turner and Down-Klinefelter syndromes. Genet Couns. 2005; 16 (4): 393-402.

[16] Ruangdaraganon N, Kotchabhakdi N, Mekanandha V. Double aneuploidy: 46,X, +21 a combination of Down syndrome and Turner syndrome. J Med Assoc Thai. 1993; 76 (2): 215-217.

[17] Glass IA, Li L, Cotter PD. Double aneuploidy (48,XXY,+21): molecular analysis demonstrates a maternal origin. Eur. J. Med. Genet 2006; 49: 346–348.

[18] Visootsak J, Graham JM. Klinefelter syndrome and other sex chromosomal aneuploidies. Orphanet. J. Rare Dis 2006; 1: 42.

[19] Akbas E, Soylemez F, Savasoglu K, Halliogluand O, Balci S. A male case with double aneuploidy (48,XXY,+21). Genet Couns. 2008;19 (1): 59-63.

[20] Yamaguchi T, Hamasuna R, Hasui Y, Kitada S, Osada Y. 47,XXY/ 48,XXY,+21 chromosomal mosaicism presenting as hypospadias with scrotal transposition. J Urol 1989; 142: 797-798.

[21] Hecht F, Nievaard JE, Duncanson N, Miller JR, Higgins JV, Kimberling WJ et al. Double aneuploidy: The frequency of XXY in males with Down syndrome. Am J Hum Genet 1969; 21: 352-359.

[22] Shen Z, Zou CC, Shang SQ and Jiang KW. Down-Klinefelter syndrome (48,XXY,+21) in a Child with Congenital Heart Disease: Case Report and Literature Review. Intern Med 2012; 51: 1371-1374.

[23] Gerretsen MF, Peelen W, Rammeloo LA, Koolbergen DR, Hruda J. Double aortic arch with double aneuploidy--rare anomaly in combined Down and Klinefelter syndrome. Eur J Pediatr. 2009; 168 (12): 1479-81.

[24] Shu X, Zou C, Shen Z. Double aneuploidy 48,XXY,+21 associated with a congenital heart defect in a neonate. BJMG 2013; 16 (2): 85-90.

[25] Iliopoulos D, Poultsides G, Peristeri V, Kouri G, Andreou A, Voyiatzis N. A Double trisomy (48,XXY,+21) in monozygotic twins: Case report and review of the literature. Ann de Genet 2004; 47: 95-98.

[26] Al Awadi SA, Naguib KK, Bastaki L, Gouda S, Mohammed F M, Abulhasan SJ et al. Down syndrome in Kuwait: Recurrent familial trisomy 21 in siblings. Downs Syndr Res Pract 1998; 5: 131-137.

[27] Hamerton J, Brigges S, Gianelli F, Carter C. Chromosomal studies in detection of parents with high risk of second child with Down's syndrome. Lancet 1961; 2: 788.

[28] Taylor AI, Moores EC. A sex chromatin survey of newborn children in two London hospitals. J Med Genet 1967; 4: 258.

[29] Mutton D, Alberman E, Hook EB. Cytogenetic and epidemiological findings in Down syndrome, England and Wales 1989 to 1993. National Down Syndrome Cytogenetic Register and the Association of Clinical Cytogeneticists. J Med Genet 1996; 33: 387–394.

[30] Kovaleva NV, Mutton DE. Epidemiology of double aneuploidies involving chromosome 21 and the sex chromosomes. Am J Med Genet A 2005; 134:24–32.

[31] Forrester MB, Merz RD. Pregnancy outcome and prenatal diagnosis of sex chromosome abnormalities in Hawaii,1986–1999. Am J Med Genet A 2003; 119:305–310.

[32] Bojesen A, Juul S, Gravholt CH. Prenatal and postnatal prevalence of Klinefelter syndrome: a national registry study. J Clin Endocrinol Metab 2003; 88: 622–626.

[33] Harnden DG, Miller OJ, Penrose LS. The Klinefeltermongolism type of double aneuploidy. Ann Hum Genet. 1960; 24: 165-169.

[34] Lanman JL, Shlarin B, Cooper H, Hirschhorn K. Klinifelter's syndrome in a ten months old mongolism idiot. N Eng J Med 1960; 263: 887.

[35] Hustinx TWJ, Eberle P, Geerts SJ, Brink JT, Woltring LM. Mongoloid twins with 48 chromosomes (AA A21XXY). Annals of Human Genetics 1961; 25: 111-113.

[36] Gelderen V and Hustinx TWJ. Combination of Klinifelter's syndrome and mongolism. Ned Tij Genetic 1961; 105: 1925-1928.

[37] Milcou M and Maianesco M. Klinifelter's syndrome associated with mongolism and bilateral testicular ectopy. Pathol Biol 1963; 11: 1247-1250.

[38] Court Brown WM, Harnden DG, Jacobs PA, Maclean N, Mantle DJ. Abnormalities of the Sex Chromosome Complement in Man. Medical Research Council 1964, Special Report No. 305. HMSO, London.

[39] Pfeiffer RA. Double aneuploidy (Trisomy 21 and XXY) in an infant. Arch Kinderheilkd. 1964;171: 69-79.

[40] Cyril C, Jagatheesan CN, Chandralekha T, Gopinath PM and Marimuthu KM. Down syndrome child with 48,XXY, +21 karyotype, Ind. J. Human. Genet 2005; 11: 47-48.

[41] Karaman A, Kabalar E. Double aneuploidy in a Turkish child: Down-Klinefelter syndrome. Congenit Anom (Kyoto). 2008; 48 (1): 45-47.

[42] Biselli JM, Machado FB, Zampieri BL, Alves da Silva AF, Goloni-Bertollo EM, Haddad R, Eberlin MN, Vannucchi H, Carvalho VM, Medina-Acosta E, Pavarino-Bertelli EC. Double aneuploidy (48,XXY,+21) of maternal origin in a child born to a 13-year-old mother: evaluation of the maternal folate metabolism. Genet Couns. 2009; 20 (3): 225-34.

[43] Jeanty C, Turner C. Prenatal Diagnosis of Double Aneuploidy, 48,XXY,+21, and Review of the Literature. Ultrasound Med 2009; 28: 673–681.

[44] Mishra SR, Bisht JS, Kumar M, Kumar S, Gaur K, Kumar R, Lal V, Bhattacharya SK. Double aneuploidy 48,XXY,+21 in a fetus with congenital abnormalities. Der Pharmacia Letter 2014; 6 (3): 351-354.

[45] Day, R. W., Wright, S. W., Koons, A., and Quigley, M. XXX 21-trisomy and retinoblastoma. Lancet 1963; 2: 154-155.

[46] Yunis JJ, Hook EB, Mayer M. DNA. replication analysis in identifying the cytogenetic defect in Down's syndrome (mongolism). Lancet. 1965; 27 (1): 465–466.

[47] Park VM, Bravo RR, Shulman LP. Double non-disjunction in maternal meiosis II giving rise to a fetus with 48,XXX,+21. J Med Genet 1995; 32: 650- 653.

[48] Devlin L, Morrison PJ. Mosaic Down's syndrome prevalence in a complete population study. Arch Dis Child. 2004; 89 (12): 1177-8.

[49] Balwan WK, Kumar P, Raina TR, Gupta S. Double trisomy with 48, XXX+21 karyotype in a Down's syndrome child from Jammu and Kashmir. Ind J Genet, 2008; 87(3): 257-259.

[50] Guzel AI, Demirhan O, Pazarbasi A, Ozgunen FT et al. Detection of parental origin and cell stage errors of a double non-disjunction in a fetus by QF-PCR. Genet Test Mol Biomarkers 2009; 13(1): 73-77.

[51] Sheth HJ, Munoz A, Sergi C, Pani J, Blouin JL, Sheth JJ, Sheth FJ. Triple-X Syndrome in a Trisomic Down Syndrome Child: Both Aneuploidies Originated from the Mother. Int J Hum Genet 2011; 11(1): 51-53.

[52] Uwineza A, Hitayezu J, Murorunkwere S, Ndinkabandi J, Mutesa L. An unusual case of double aneuploidy of down syndrome associated with triple X syndrome: 48,XXX, +21. Rwanda Medical Journal 2012; 69 (4): 27-29.

[53] Verresen, H. and van den Berghe, H. 21-trisomy and XYY. Lancet 1965; 1: 609.

[54] Migeon BR. G trisomy in an XYY male. Human Chromosome Newsletter 1965; 17: 16.

[55] Uchida, I. A., Ray, M., and Duncan, B. P. 21 Trisomy with an XYY sex chromosome complement. Journal of Pediatrics 1966; 69: 295-298.

[56] Al-Aish MS, Dodson WE, Plato CC. Down's syndrome with XYY: 48,XYY, G+. Am J Dis Child. 1971; 121 (5): 444-446.

[57] Schwanitz G, Hagner M. Double trisomy as a mosaic. Case history (48, XYY, +21/47, XY, +21) and survey of the literature of mixed autosomal-gonosomal trisomies. Acta Genet Med Gemellol (Roma) 1978; 27: 67–74.

[58] Reddy KS. Double trisomy in spontaneous abortions. Hum Genet. 1997;101 (3): 339-45.

[59] Parmar RC' Muranjan MN, Swami S. Trisomy 21 with XYY. Indian J Pediatr. 2002; 69 (11): 979-981.

[60] Koken R, Bukulmez A. Double Aneuploidy: A Case of Trisomy 21 with XYY. Eur J Gen Med 2011; 8 (4): 338-341.

[61] Parihar M, Koshy B, Srivastava VM. Mosaic double aneuploidy: Down syndrome and XYY. Indian J Hum Genet. 2013; 19(3): 346–348.

[62] Lorda-Sanchez I, Petersen MB, Binkert F, Maechler M, Schmid W, Adelsberger PA et al. A 48,XXY,+21 Down syndrome patient with additional paternal X and maternal 21. Hum Genet 1991; 87: 54-56.

[63] Subramaniyam S, Pulijaal VR, Mathew S. Double and multiple chromosomal aneuploidies in spontaneous abortions: A single institutional experience. Journal of Human Reproductive Sciences 2014; 7 (4): 262-263.

[64] Caron L, Tihy F, Dallaire L. Frequencies of chromosomal abnormalities at amniocentesis: over 20 years of cytogenetic analyses in one laboratory. Am J Med Genet 1999; 82: 149–154.

[65] Oliver TR, Feingold E, Yu K, Cheung V, Tinker S, et al. New insights into human nondisjunction of chromosome 21 in oocytes. PLoS Genet 2008; 4 (3): 1-9.